Herniated Spinal Discs Absorb Better

The Truth about Herniated Discs

Herniated Spinal Discs Absorb Better

1st Edition Printed | December 1, 2020
1st Edition Issued | December 10, 2020

Author	Jaseng Hospital of Korean Medicine · Jaseng Spine and Joint Research Institute
Planned and Translated by	Jaseng Medical Academy
Edited by	Joseph Queeney
Website	jaseng.education

Publisher	Ju-Yeun Chang
Editing Design by	Eun-jung Yang
Cover Design by	Jae-wook Kim
Produced by	Sang-hyeon Shin
Publishing House	Koonja Publishing, Inc.
	Registration No. 4-139 (June 24, 1991)
	Paju Publishing Complex, 338, Hoedong-gil (474-1 Seopae-dong),
	Paju-si, Gyeonggi-do, South Korea (10881)
	Telephone: (031) 943-1888 Fax: (031) 955-9545
	Website: www.koonja.co.kr

ISBN 979-11-5955-625-8

CONTENTS

CHAPTER **2** What Causes Herniated Discs?

CONTENTS

CHAPTER **4** Herniated Spinal Discs Absorb Better

CONTENTS

CHAPTER 6 Nine Small But Important Questions Asked by Herniated Disc Patients

Restoring the Self-Healing Power of the Spine through Scientifically-Proven Korean Medicine

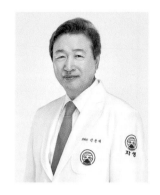

Since its establishment in 1988, Jaseng Hospital of Korean Medicine has helped many patients unable to move from extreme pain due to severe disc herniation and nerve root compression recover and return to their everyday lives.

The intervertebral disc consists of the nucleus pulposus and annulus fibrosus with innervation to the outer portion of the annulus fibrosus, and thus the disc does not feel pain by itself. However, under excessive external force, the annulus fibrosus is no longer able to contain the nucleus pulposus, and the disrupted or extruded nucleus pulposus may compress the nerve root, incurring extreme pain. In cases of disc extrusion, non-invasive Korean medicine treatment may be more effective than surgery for swift pain reduction and improvement of self-healing power by strengthening the spine, joint, and nerve structures.

Self-healing power refers to the body's ability to recover spontaneously from illness. It refers to the innate ability and power that helps us return to health when our body is sick or out of balance. It is easy to understand if you think of how the body heals itself if you give an injury wound time to recover after cleansing, or a fractured bone held in a cast.

Jaseng Hospital of Korean Medicine uses non-invasive treatments that employ an integrative medicine approach – comprising of conventional and

Korean medicine – which determines the patient's current condition using X-rays, MRIs, and blood tests, and strengthens and regenerates weakened bones and nerves to treat the fundamental cause of disorders, as opposed to temporary pain relief. As such, optimal evidence-based treatments are used to the aim of strengthening the body's overall resilience and preventing recurrence.

The effects and safety of Jaseng treatments, including "Shinbaro herbal medicine," the main herbal medicine used at Jaseng, "Motion Style Acupuncture Treatment (MSAT)," and "Chuna Manual Therapy", have been scientifically proven through research and papers published in collaboration with leading researchers affiliated with various world renowned national and international universities. Today, physicians from medical institutions around the world including the U.S., Russia, Kazakhstan and the Middle East come to our hospital to study our techniques.

This book covers not only Jaseng's treatments for herniated disc, but also personal stories from our doctors and patients. I hope that more medical staff and patients may become knowledgeable of Jaseng's treatments, and that this knowledge may help them regain their self-healing power through non-invasive treatments rather than surgery to lead happier, healthier lives.

Jaseng Hospital of Korean Medicine will continue to work with commitment to contributing to the betterment of the health of mankind with such distinguished partners as Arkansas Colleges of Health Education (ACHE).

Dr. Joon-Shik Shin, KMD, Ph.D., S.D.
Jaseng Hospital of Korean Medicine

서문

과학적 한방 치료로
허리의 자생력을 되살린다

자생한방병원은 1988년 개원이래 디스크가 터져서 흘러나오고, 신경을 압박하고 있는 중증디스크로 인하여 자리에서 일어나지 못하고 극심한 통증을 호소하는 수많은 환자들을 일상으로 돌아가도록 도와주었다.

디스크는 수핵과 수핵을 둘러싸고있는 섬유륜만으로 이루어져있어 그 자체로는 통증을 느끼지 못한다. 하지만 외부의 과도한 힘을 받으면, 수핵을 둘러싸고 있는 섬유륜이 더 이상 버티지 못하고 밀려나가거나 터져 신경근을 압박하여 극심한 통증이 발생된다.
디스크가 터진 경우 수술보다 비수술 한방치료를하면 빠른 통증 감소와 더불어 척추 뼈와 관절, 신경이 강화되어 자생력이 강화되는 효과가 있다.

자생력이란, 스스로 자신의 질병을 치유하는 능력을 말한다. 우리 몸이 질병에 걸렸거나 균형을 잃었을 때, 이를 회복하게 도와주는 힘이다.
상처가 났을 때 그대로 두면 자연스럽게 아물고, 뼈에 금이 갔을 때 깁스로 고정해주면 일정시간 경과 후 회복되는 것을 생각하면 이해하기 쉽다.

자생한방병원은 "비수술"을 내세워 일시적으로 통증을 줄이는 치료법이 아닌 한양방의 협진을 통하여 X-ray, MRI, 혈액검사 등으로 정확한 상태를 파악하고, 손상된 뼈와 신경을 재생시켜 질환의 원인을 근본적으로 바로잡는다. 약해진 인체를 강화시켜 재발방지까지 하는 가장 안전하고 과학적인 치료법을 시행한다고 할 수 있다.

자생한방병원의 대표적 한약인 "신바로 한약"과 "동작침법", "추나요법"을 포함한 여러 치료법은 국내외 유수의 대학 연구진과 함께 논문을 통해 과학적으로 증명되었고, 현재는 미국, 러시아, 카자흐스탄, 중동 등 해외에서도 자생의 치료법을 배우고 있다.

이 책에는 자생의 디스크 치료법뿐만 아니라 자생의 한의사와 환자들의 이야기도 함께 담겨있다. 많은 의료진과 환자들이 자생의 치료법을 알고, 수술보다는 비수술 치료법으로 스스로의 자생력을 되찾아 건강한 삶을 이어가길 바란다.

앞으로도 자생한방병원은 미국 아칸소 보건교육대학(ACHE) 등 세계 유수의 협력 기관들과 함께 인류의 건강증진 기여에 힘쓸 수 있도록 사명감을 갖고 꾸준히 노력할 것이다.

신준식, 자생한방병원   신 준 식

Three Questions and Three Prejudices that Herniated Disc Patients Carry

"Can my condition be cured without surgery?" "Can Korean medicine completely cure my condition?" "Why did my discs herniate?" These are some of the several questions that patients suffering from herniated discs ask during consultations.

These kinds of questions stem from three main prejudices. The first is the belief that herniated discs can be treated only with surgery; the second is the presumption that conventional medicine provides the only treatment option; and the last is the assumption that their own discs will not rupture.

Herniated discs can be treated without surgery. To go even further, I claim that they must be treated without surgery. Some patients visit my clinic when their herniated disc conditions recur after undergoing back surgery. When I, having examined their X-ray images, ask if they have previously undergone back surgery, many patients are surprised that I am able to accurately determine their medical histories. In most herniated spinal disc surgeries, the surgeon makes an incision on the skin and muscles and removes a portion of the spinal bones. This enables them to see the nerves, which are then retracted in order to bring the extruded discs into view. It is only after this process that the extruded discs can be dissected. This also means that most patients who undergo back surgery for their herniated discs do not have all the parts of their spinal bones fully intact.

Because X-ray images show the patients' bones, they often indicate the interventions applied during surgery. The majority of patients are unaware that parts of their bones were removed during their back surgery. They are usually under the impression that their operation was a simple one.

Surgery, however, irreversibly change and damage to the body. Herniated discs are caused by a weakening of the back and spine. When surgeons make incisions into the muscles and ligaments to cut away damaged discs, they only worsen the stability of these structures. In many cases, bones are also damaged during operative procedures. To be clear, surgery is indeed required for some herniated disc patients, but such patients make up less than five percent of all individuals diagnosed with herniated discs. Statistics, however, show that doctors recommend back surgery to an overwhelming proportion of herniated disc patients, many of whom eventually do agree to undergo surgery.

So, can herniated discs be completely cured with Korean medicine? To answer this question, we must understand the definition of "completely cured". If we decide to define "completely cured" as restoring a dried and flattened disc to its previous plump, elastic, liquid-filled states, or if "normal" allows the patients to continue bad habits that damaged the discs while preventing recurrence of herniation indefinitely, neither alternative nor conventional medicine treatments can return a herniated disc back to "normal". On the other hand, if the definition of "complete cured" as the state of ruptured discs that naturally absorb back with significantly reduced pain, and help patients improve their posture and habits that could cause recurrence of herniation, then there is a high chance that herniated discs can be "completely cured."

Surgical treatments, analgesics, and steroids have served as an efficient means by which to manage problems associated with protruded discs.

Simply put, the extruding portion of the discs was removed, and pain was alleviated through medication. On the other hand, Korean medicine focuses on factors that caused the discs to herniate in the first place. Korean medicine doctors use combinations of herbal medicine ingredients that strengthen the muscles and bones (as stated in the traditional Korean medical book Dongeui Bogam), in addition to Chuna manual therapy that aims to correct the posture and fix the unique, fundamental issues that contribute to the individual patient's herniated disc condition.

When patients ask why their discs are ruptured, what they are really asking is why they are one of only a few people who suffer from the condition. Such sentiment is more prevalent in those who are born with a weaker back, those who have narrower lumbar arteries that deliver nutrition to the back, and those with a congenitally improper spinal skeletal alignment. The levels of pain sensitivity for those experiencing this condition are widely diverse. Some individuals hardly feel any pain despite a severe disc herniation, while others are rushed to the emergency room with even a slight swelling in their discs.

Despite the fact that pain is often the most prominent and supposedly urgent effect of herniated discs that patients complain about, medical professionals at Jaseng attempt to look beyond just the area of pain. They seek to target the cause of the condition, particularly by correcting patients' lifestyles and other external or internal factors. In the past, when the expected lifespan of humans was much shorter, there were most likely less issues associated with herniated discs. Yet as the expected lifespan becomes longer and longer and people live to become older and older, people who have habits or other influences that contribute to the weakening of their discs will inevitably suffer from spinal diseases at some point in their lives. Without solving the fundamental issues associated with these diseases, such patients will have to suffer for many more years to come.

Every patient who walks into my office is told what I have just mentioned above. Before starting treatment for patients whose pain sometimes prevents them even from sitting, I ensure that they fully understand what a disc herniation is. I believe that a patient's clear understanding of their disease or condition plays a large role in their future attitude towards it. Many patients, however, are poorly educated about their condition from medical professionals, which distorts their perception about herniated discs. This further exacerbates their situation. I hope this book will impart necessary knowledge to patients about their condition, while also becoming a source of advice and encouragement to help them overcome their condition.

Dr. In-Hyuk Ha, KMD, Ph.D.

Director of Jaseng Spine and Joint Research Institute

ACKNOWLEDGEMENT

The publication of the newly translated edition of Herniated Spinal Discs Absorb Better, edited by Joseph Queeney, DO, FACOS, faculty at Arkansas College of Osteopathic Medicine (ARCOM) exemplifies a collaborative effort in cross-cultural, interprofessional understanding of how Western medicine and Korean traditional medicine may be integrated. Here, assisted by Donald Sefcik, DO, MBA, Assistant Dean of Clinical Medicine, and Student Doctor David Kim, OMS-1, Dr. Queeney has captured the essence of the original Korean language edition.

With great pride of ARCOM's participation in this book, I congratulate Jaseng Hospital of Korean Medicine in its effort to bring to the world what Jaseng has been practicing for more than 30 years. I look forward to further collaboration with Jaseng.

Brian G. Kim, J.D.

President, Arkansas Colleges of Health Education (ACHE)

PROLOGUE

Herniated Discs Can Be Completely Cured with Non-Invasive Korean Medicine Treatment

"You can fix my herniated discs without surgery, can't you?" Many patients who wish desperately to avoid undergoing surgery often visit Jaseng Hospital of Korean Medicine. They commonly ask this question because of their aversion to surgery. They want confirmation that non-invasive treatments – Korean medicine treatments in particular – can cure herniated discs. Of course, such questions that betray mixed feelings of anxiety and hope are understandable, considering that most of them have already visited a doctor practicing conventional medicine who recommended surgery. Our approach of non-invasive treatment, however, is completely different.

It is difficult to believe in something that one has not experienced or witnessed firsthand. One thing is for certain, though: countless patients with herniated discs have come to Jaseng Hospital of Korean Medicine, and have directly experienced how non-invasive treatments have completely improved their conditions. In addition to acute disc herniation patients, even chronic disc herniation patients have reported rapid health recovery, and are now leading pain-free lives.

It has taken quite a while to prove that herniated discs can be cured exclusively with Korean medicine non-invasive treatments, without any forms of invasive surgery. Despite numerous cases of patients, who could not even walk prior to treatment, experiencing immediate improvement after undergoing herbal medicine, Chuna manual therapy, Motion Style Acupuncture Treatment, and pharmacopuncture, the spinal medicine community did not so easily recognize the effectiveness of Korean medicine non-invasive treatments. As such, my team and I devoted extensive time and energy to scientifically prove the mechanisms of our methods. As a result, no one in the spinal medicine community today disputes the effectiveness of Korean medicine non-invasive treatments.

Herniated discs are not caused overnight. Some patients claim that their discs suddenly ruptured and induced pain because they were lifting heavy objects or quickly changing postures. This is not true. Discs gradually weaken due to several factors, including aging, lack of nutrition, and adverse life habits. Discs can weaken without any knowledge of the patient, and they rupture when a sudden and excessive shock is applied. There is not a single case in which normal, healthy discs suddenly rupture out of the blue.

As such, herniated or ruptured discs indicate that the related organs have already been significantly weakened. This means that ruptured discs especially require non-invasive treatment, as opposed to surgery. During surgery, extruded discs are cut out. This process can damage the muscles and ligaments that surround the discs; in some cases, spinal bones are drilled, which often further damages the already weakened discs. Patients may be misled into thinking that they have been cured because they feel less pressure on their nerves is released, which removes the source of pain. However, the truth is that their backs have been structurally compromised through such back surgeries.

Unlike invasive operations, Korean medicine non-invasive treatments seek to make full use of the self-healing power within the spinal bones and discs. These methods quickly and effectively eliminate the pain caused by herniated discs while simultaneously fortifying the self-healing power of the human body. The treatments remove the cause of herniated or ruptured discs and prevent recurrences at the same time.

Korean medicine non-invasive treatments are highly effective ways to heal herniated discs on a fundamental level. Complete recovery, however, is difficult when using exclusively non-invasive methods.

Since herniated discs require continued management of conditions, neglecting general maintenance of health after the symptoms have been alleviated will cause the discs to herniate or rupture again. For example, a patient whose discs ruptured due to a lifestyle that puts excessive pressure on his back will have a high risk of recurrence if he resumes his previous lifestyle, even after the conditions have improved through non-invasive treatments.

Patients need not worry too much since discs that rupture again can be healed with Korean medicine non-invasive treatments. However, to prevent future pain induced by the relapse of herniated discs, patients should take the time, while undergoing non-invasive treatment, to reflect upon their lifestyles and habits. They must think about what led to their conditions in the first place, change their lifestyles to prevent further suffering and take a step towards completely curing their herniated discs.

1

The Surprising Truth
About Herniated Discs

1. Do You Need Surgery for Herniated Discs?

Surgery Is Not the Only Answer to Herniated Discs

"Do you really think it will really be okay? Do I need surgery for a ruptured discs? Can I really be cured without surgery?" These are common questions asked by patients who visit our hospital for ruptured discs. Even though they come to Jaseng because of their aversion to and reluctance towards surgery, they are not fully aware of the healing power used in non-invasive treatments. This indicates the deeply embedded misconception that surgery is the only solution for ruptured or herniated discs.

In fact, it has not been too long since it was proven that ruptured discs can be treated without surgery. A fascinating study concerning treatment of ruptured discs was published in 1983, challenging the conventionally held beliefs about disc surgery.

The study, frequently cited in the spine medical research community to this day, was conducted by Swedish doctor, Dr. Henrik Weber.

In this study, Dr. Weber randomly assigned 126 herniated disc patients to two groups: a control group that received surgery, and another that received other treatments. The progress of these patients was tracked, compared, and studied over the course of ten years. The research results were published in an article titled "Lumbar Disc Herniation: A Controlled, Prospective Study with Ten Years of Observation." The findings are as follows:

In Weber's study, the patients in one group received surgery for their herniated discs, and the patients in the other group received non-invasive treatments, including physical therapy and pharmacologic therapy. At first, the group of patients who received surgery seemed to show better progess because their pain dissipated more quickly. After four years, however, the disc conditions of the patients between the two groups were not very different.

The results of Weber's study shocked the surgical spine community that had believed that surgery was the only answer to herniated discs. This questioned the belief of many medical practitioners, who had previously believed that surgery was an inevitable solution. As more doctors carefully considered the study, which reported that surgery did not have vastly different results compared to non-surgical treatments, the opinions of the medical community began to shift. New guidelines were established. Rather than immediately operating on disc herniation patients, doctors were advised to incorporate two to three months of non-invasive treatments, observe any progress, and then make decisions regarding surgery.

Before Treatment

After Treatment

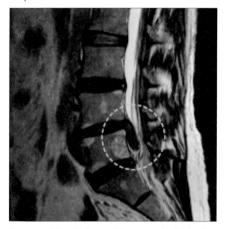
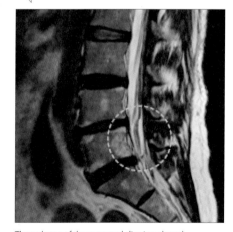

A ruptured disc is observed between the L4 lumbar spine and L5 lumbar spine

The volume of the ruptured disc is reduced.

These are photos of a forty-three-year-old woman with a ruptured disc before and after receiving treatment. The patient's ruptured disc was healed with just Korean medicine treatments, without surgery.

Despite these changes, lumbar spinal surgeries are still prevalent in Korea, both because medical professionals are not able to control initial pain with non-invasive treatments, and because of the lack of certainty and experience regarding such non-surgical options. Jaseng Hospital of Korean Medicine, however, has been treating herniated discs through non-invasive means for more than thirty years. This was before the majority of hospitals were familiar about the use and effects of such methods. Through numerous clinical cases, Jaseng has proven that non-invasive treatment methods can effectively reduce pain during the early stages of the disease, in addition to successfully curing it without surgery.

Because of the long-term, tireless efforts by Jaseng, now Korean hospitals are less likely to perform surgery for herniated discs. Even conventional medicine hospitals tend to seek out non-invasive treatments prior to surgery. Quite a few hospitals, however, still recommend and advocate surgery for their patients throughout the entire process.

Through the experience of Jaseng, which has been treating herniated discs with non-invasive methods for over thirty years, there are not many patients who will ultimately require surgery. Ninety-five percent of herniated disc patients can be cured by only non-invasive treatments, and, in many cases, with better results than if surgery had been performed. Furthermore, patients report higher satisfaction for non-invasive treatments than for surgery, and say that the former is more effective.

Common Misconceptions About Different Types of Paralyses

Even when discs are ruptured, non-invasive methods can effectively treat the condition. Even when the discs are completely ruptured, causing extreme pain, non-invasive treatments administered at Jaseng Hospital can more reliably eliminate pain than surgery. There are countless cases in which patients have fully recovered and can return to their normal, everyday lives.

There are, however, some cases in which surgery is necessary. If a ruptured discs is

Ruptured Disc?

Many herniated disc patients often say that their discs are "ruptured." Medically, a "ruptured disc" refers to the tearing of the annulus fibrosus, which causes the nucleus pulposus to extrude beyond its normal position. Indicating that it is a state in which the disc is extruded. Patients broadly refer to this condition as their discs having been "ruptured."

Discs generally do not extrude when disc herniation first occurs. At first, the disc is usually only slightly herniated or in a bulging state, and does not extensively compress the nerves. The pain may still be great at this stage. When the condition progresses further, however, the nucleus pulposus extrudes beyond the outer borders of the annulus fibrosus, and may compress the spinal cord or nerve roots. This stage is termed disc protrusion. At this stage, the annulus fibrosus, though weakened, is mainly still intact, preventing the nucleus pulposus from herniating extensively.

When patients say that their discs are "torn," their discs may actually be extruded or protruded. Based on the shape of the displaced disc material, herniated discs may be classified as protrusion or extrusion. Although extrusion and protrusion are different stages of disc herniation, it is sometimes difficult to differentiate between the two stages on imaging test results. Also, for general practice, differentiating whether disc rupture refers to disc extrusion or protrusion is generally not of critical importance clinically. This book also refers to disc herniation as disc "rupture" regardless of whether the discs are protruded or extruded, with the nucleus pulposus extensively displaced, inflammation and irritation, or compression of the nerves to incur pain.

pressing down on the cauda equina, a spinal nerve bundle that controls their bladder and bowel, the patient may become incontinent. This is an emergent situation that requires immediate surgery within three days. If surgery is not performed emergently, this condition could become permanent and irreversible.

In that case, do all paralytic symptoms require surgery? Quite a few patients visit Jaseng Hospital of Korean Medicine for recurring herniated disc symptoms after receiving surgery at another medical institution. They say things like: "I had herniated disc surgery ten years ago. I've been doing well since then, but I started experiencing pain again recently."

If the patient did not experience any pain for ten years following the surgery, the back should have remained in a relatively healthy state. If the patient underwent surgery when the back was weak, it would have been difficult for the patient to be pain free for ten years. This also means that the patient would have been able to recover without surgery ten years ago.

I asked this particular patient, "It doesn't seem that your back condition warranted surgery. Why did you agree to the operation?" She answered, "I had paralysis back then, therefore I had to do the surgery."

It is natural to consider surgery inevitable when facing paralysis. The paralysis that patients think of is not due to loss of neurologic function, it is an inability of move secondary to the back pain.

Patients often say, "I was scared when I couldn't move all of a sudden. I was afraid of being bedridden for the rest of my life, so I called emergency health services to go to the hospital."

In the past, nine out of ten of such patients would have undergone surgery. With patients scared about their conditions and futures, they almost always strictly followed the doctors' recommendations for surgery.

Many patients also come to Jaseng with acute paralytic symptoms. When they cannot move their bodies, patients experience extreme fear. It is rare, however, that such paralytic patients require emergency surgery.

Patients with paralysis then ask, "Why can I not move my body at all, then? Is my condition so bad that I need surgery?" When patients experience severe symptoms and pain, they will often disagree with their doctors who tell them that their herniated discs are not very severe. Stiffness and severe pain the natural ways of protecting itself. When discs rupture to press down on the nerves and cause acute pain, the body recognizes this as an emergency and engages defensive mechanisms to protect the discs.

Since discs can suffer further damage if the related muscles continue to be used, the brain halts the movements of the muscles. This results in the muscles surrounding the discs to stiffen, thereby preventing muscle movement and causing patients to think that they are paralyzed.

Such temporary "paralysis" occurs to protect the discs are not symptoms that indicate the need for surgery. Many patients who are admitted to our hospital in a stiffened state walk out the door recovered and healthy after a couple of days of non-invasive Korean medicine treatment. The paralysis that patients experience when their discs first rupture is often due to extreme pain.

Motion Style Acupuncture Treatment, a non-invasive treatment, can quickly eliminate the pain. When the pain subsides as a result of Motion Style Acupuncture Treatment, the brain disengages from its protective state. The stiffened muscles are allowed to relax, thereby alleviating the "paralysis."

Surgery must be performed when necessary, but temporary paralytic symptoms should not automatically trigger the need for surgery. It is important to closely examine whether the patient's current condition truly requires surgery or not. Paralytic symptoms that indicate need for surgery include bowel and bladder dysfunction and progressive loss of neurological function(i.e., when the patient cannot elevate their legs against resistance). Conducting surgery simply because of stiffness can actually worsen the situation.

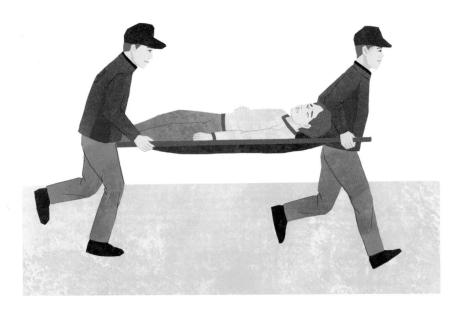

2. Do Degrees of Disc Herniation and Pain Level Match?

Does the Lack of Pain Mean You're Cured?

Few people go to see the doctor when they are not experiencing back pain. Most visit a hospital when their back hurts. Patients go to the doctor for a wide range of reasons, from the pain associated with spraining a back to chronic back pain, and even the inability to walk.

Since most patients seek medical assistance to treat pain, many mistakes the lack of pain as an indication that their condition has been cured. It is dangerous to assume that no more treatment is required when there is no pain. This is because the degree of severity of disc herniation or disc rupture and the level of pain often do not correspond with each other. There may not be any pain associated with a highly severe case of disc rupture, and there may be intense pain without severe herniation. To understand this phenomenon, we must first examine the process by which discs rupture and induce pain.

Discs consist of a soft and plump central nucleus pulposus and the surrounding annulus fibrosus, which is tough and elastic. The nucleus pulposus normally sits at the center of the disc, like the yolk of an egg. When the nucleus pulposus pushes through the annulus fibrosus for some reason, it extrudes and presses down on the nerves resulting in pain. The situation can further worsen, if the disc ruptures and the nucleus pulposus leaks out.

A simple extrusion of the nucleus pulposus without a disc rupture is serious enough; rupturing and leaking are indications of an urgent problem. The leaking nucleus pulposus pressing down on the spinal nerves induces pain. It consequently causes the swelling and inflammation of the spinal nerve thereby exacerbating the pain.

Disc ruptures are not necessarily accompanied by severe pain. Depending on the direction of the disc rupture, the patient may experience different types of pain, or no pain at all.

When the nucleus pulposus protrudes in the middle, where there is more space between the nerves, it does not press down on the enerve roots rven (which controls the legs) very much. This means that the patient will experience primarily back pain. On the other hand, if the nucleus pulposus extrudes to the left or right, where the nerves are more densely packed, it can press down on the nerve roots, causing more pain in the legs than in the back. Many patients complain that their "back disc herniation" is causing more pain in the legs than in the back. This is because the disc has ruptured, causing the nucleus pulposus to press down on the nerve roots that control the legs.

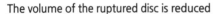

The volume of the ruptured disc is reduced

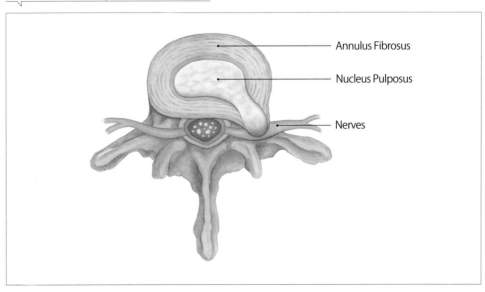

Annulus Fibrosus

Nucleus Pulposus

Nerves

In general, it is easy for discs to rupture posterolaterally, near the spinal nerves. This is because the lumbar spine tends to bend forward rather than backward in everyday movements, putting more pressure on the backside of the discs. Occasionally, however, discs may rupture on the front side. In such cases, patients may not experience pain at all, since nerves do not pass anterior to the abdominal side of the discs.

Also, even when the discs are ruptured, there may be minimal pain if a small portion of the nucleus pulposus has leaked out. This is because the spaces around discs are

Normal Discs

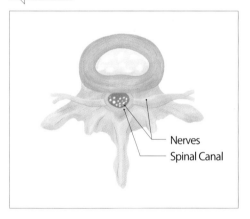

Nerves

Spinal Canal

If the discs are ruptured in the middle and the nerves are not pressed down

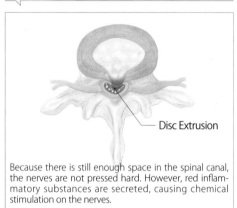

Disc Extrusion

Because there is still enough space in the spinal canal, the nerves are not pressed hard. However, red inflammatory substances are secreted, causing chemical stimulation on the nerves.

In case the spinal canal is congenitally narrow and the nerves are pressed down even with a small rupture on the discs

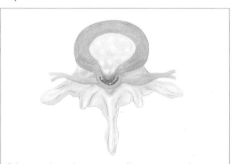

If the spinal canal is congenitally narrow, or it becomes narrow due to degenerative changes, pain becomes more severe because discs press down on the nerves in a narrower space

When the discs are ruptured towards a narrow space to severely press down on the nerves

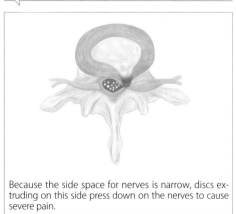

Because the side space for nerves is narrow, discs extruding on this side press down on the nerves to cause severe pain.

quite large: ruptured discs do not immediately compress the spinal nerves. If there is pain even when the rupture is not serious, it is due to the inflammation of the torn annulus fibrosus. Also, even when the nucleus pulposus does not compress the nerves, it may leak out and chemically inflame the nerves and result in pain.

As explained, there are many reasons for pain, and the severity of the pain and the severity of disc herniation rarely correlate. Nevertheless, many patients choose to stop receiving treatment, sometimes even before completing the recommended regimen, because they do not experience pain anymore.

If the root cause of the herniated disc persists, the condition will continue to progress even when the pain has resolved. The nucleus pulposus can continue to leak through the weakened annulus fibrosus. The pressure on the nerves increasesand the pain returns.If the patient were to resume treatment and the pain subsides, the herniated disc condition may worsen even more during the repeated process, ultimately causing severe pain that is worse that the initial symptoms. The treatment plan should be base on the state of the herniated discand not on the patients pain level. That is the only way to escape from the vicious cycle of recurrence and exacerbation of the condition.

People experience pain differently

Even with the same degree of disc rupture, some patients report tremendous pain, while others hardly feel any pain at all. This is not because the direction of the rupture or the amount of the leaking nucleus pulposus is different; rather, it is simply because of differing degrees of paintolerance.

Some people are more sensitive to pain than others. Those with higher sensitivity are more prone to inflammation, and others have more sensitive nerves. Such patients experience extreme pain even for relatively less severe disc herniation.

From a doctor's perspective, however, it is easier to treat patients who are more sensitive to pain. This is because patients who are not as sensitive to pain or inaccurately report pain in the wrong part of the body often do not understand the severity of the condition, which makes them underestimate the appropriate timing for treatment.

Patients who are less sensitive to pain often come to my hospital and say that they wish to have their backs examined because of dull soreness. They say, "My back was sore sometimes, but I've never felt much pain. I came just to have my back looked at."

They confidently talk about their condition as they undergo examinations, which frequently reveal aggravating conditions. Because they did not experience extreme pain in their backs, they do not realize that their discs have ruptured quite severely, and are now pressing down on the nerves. Unless the condition is severely acute and accompanied by injury, the discs do not generally extrude at once. The condition gradually progresses by a few millimeters every year. Because the process is so gradual, people who are less sensitive to pain do not feel that their discs are herniating. When the discs begin to press down on the nerves more firmly at a later stage, such patients finally experience extreme pain, leading them to rush to a hospital.

On the other hand, some patients are carried into the hospital on a stretcher, claiming that their discs are severely herniated or ruptured. After thoroughly examining such patients, I often find that their conditions are not as serious as expected. Such patients are more sensitive to inflammation of the nerves surrounding the herniated discs. Even with a mild form of disc herniation, they may be experiencing a higher degree of pain that prevents them from moving. They usually respond well to treatment and recover more quickly. However, such patients who focus only on the acute pain may not pay attention to preventing the long-term progression of their herniated discs only to return to the hospital on a stretcher.

In the early stages of disc herniation, the discs are not extensively damaged, making treatment for both the condition and the pain easier. When the condition has progressed, the discs have been greatly damaged, making recovery more difficult and leaving long term aftereffects.

Under no circumstances should there be an attempt at correlating the degree of pain and the progress of the disc herniation. There is no reason to immediately seek medical attention because of a single episode of severe pain. However, if the pain is persistent or frequent, the patient should seek medical attention and possible diagnostic testing to investigate a possible disc herniation. Rather than just thinking that they will be fine, patients should seek medical help to have their backs examined and identify their conditions accurately. The key to maintaining healthy discs is to follow expert advice and receive appropriate treatments.

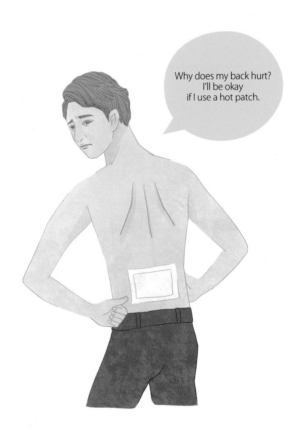

3. Are Herniated Discs Naturally Absorbed Without Intervention?

Natural Healing Is More Than a Hope: It's a Reality

Can ruptured discs be naturally absorbed without intervention? For ruptured disc patients whose treatments have only temporary effects and their recurring conditions continue to induce pain, this may sound like an unachievable fantasy. Of course, it is hard to believe that a condition that will not go away even with intensive treatment can be eliminated without much intervention.

It is, however, not a fantasy. It has been medically proven that ruptured discs can be absorbed even without surgery. A study by Dr. Komori from Japan provides compelling evidence for this. The researcher worked with 77 herniated disc patients suffering from back pain. An MRI scan was performed immediately These were compared to a second series of scans performed several months later for comparison No subjects underwent surgery or received pain reduction treatments.

The results were striking. Among the 77 patients, the size of the extruded discs naturally reduced in 49 patients (63.7% of the total subjects). Even more remarkable was the fact that in 10 out of 77 patients (13% of the total subjects), the extruded discs returned to their healthy, original states with no intervention whatsoever.

The extrusion of discs is the very last stage of disc herniation and indicates that the situation is dire for the patient. The results of Dr. Komori's research demonstrated that the majority of patients were able to recover without the need for surgery. These findings were remarkable because most doctors believed that surgery was the only option.

This is also true for the patients who are treated at Jaseng Hospital of Korean Medicine show that herniated back discs can be healed naturally. It is common for patients with pain that prevented them from even walking normally to have much smaller or even entirely eliminated protruded or extruded discs demonstrated on MRI scans performed several months later.

Some people do not believe in the power of natural healing despite these facts. Not all patients with disc abnormalities can be 100% naturally healed. In rare cases, omitting herniated disc intervention can worsen the symptoms and pain. Over time these patients spend substantial amounts of money to successfully treat their pain.

Most spinal disc herniation patients, however, improve over time. Even patients whose conditions appear less responsive and do not show natural spontaneous recovery at first hold potent self-healing properties. Rather, their conditions worsen because they, out of their lack of understanding of natural healing, undergo invasive treatments. Trusting our bodies' self-healing power and allowing the body to work of its own accord can significantly improve herniated disc conditions.

How Do Extruded Discs Heal Themselves?

How can extruded discs heal naturally when they are not surgically removed? Our bodies can, in fact, heal themselves. This is called self-healing power, or natural healing power. This natural ability of the body also comes into play when treating disc herniation.

When we say that the extruded discs are gone, it means that the nucleus pulposus that had leaked out of the ruptured annulus fibrosus has been reabsorbed. Understanding the process in which the nucleus pulposus is reabsorbed will help understand how self-healing is possible for herniated discs.

Our bodies have macrophages that consume harmful bacteria, viruses, inflammatory cells, foreign substances, and other substances that may cause diseases. These macrophages help the body maintain good health despite the constant invasion of pathogens.

When discs protrude or rupture and press down on the nerves, the macrophages immediately go into battle mode. They consider the nucleus pulposus that is leaking from the discs as a dangerous enemy and begin to consume it indiscriminately. This reduces the amount of leaked nucleus pulposus and reduces the size of the disc pressing compressing the nerves.

Even when the discs are simply protruding, the macrophages will try to consume the portion that is tprotruding. However, the annulus fibrosus that wraps around the nucleus pulposus makes it difficult for the macrophages to do so. This is why ruptured and extruded discs are more easily reabsorbed. When the annulus fibrosus is ruptured, it leaves the macrophages free to consume the softer nucleus pulposus. When the tougher annulus fibrosus is in the way, however, it inhibits the function of the macrophages, thereby prolonging the time it takes for the protruded disc to be reabsorbed into the body.

In any case, both protruded and extruded discs can be reabsorbed, despite the variation in the time required for the processes. Thus, surgery or other invasive procedures to remove the protruding discs are not required, as the body will self-heal. As such, patients suffering from severe pain due to their disc disease should not make a hasty decision to undergo surgery. Instead, they should give their bodies sufficient time to self-heal the damaged discs.

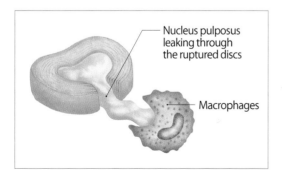

Nucleus pulposus
leaking through
the ruptured discs

Macrophages

Treatments Are Required for Natural Healing

One thing must be clarified before we move on. Many patients think that leaving the disc to self-heal means that no treatment whatsoever required, and time alone will allow for the natural healing process to take place. This is not true. Because disc herniation is accompanied by severe pain in most cases, patients suffering from this condition cannot be just left to suffer on their own. The patients' bodies will be able to deal with the condition only when the pain is alleviated.

Conventional medicine and Korean medicine have different ways of reducing pain. To relieve pain, conventional medicine uses physical therapy or potent analgesics, or steroids. In many cases, however, such treatments are ineffective. In addition to being largely ineffective, some of these treatments can actually damage discovery time.

A study regarding steroid injections in knee cartilage, a structure similar to spinal discs, was recently published in the New England Journal of Medicine (NEJM), a world-renowned medical journal. The research team studied two different groups of subjects, the control group was administered potent steroids, and the other group was injected with sterile water. The injections were given 9 times over a span of 2 years. Both groups of patients reported similar levels of knee pain following treatment.

The problem was the rate at which cartilage damage progressed. Theoretically, the anti-inflammatory properties of the steroids should have healed the damaged cartilages and slowed down the rate at which they deteriorated. Yet during the 2 years of the study, the joint cartilage deterioration was greater in the group that was administered steroids.

The group that received steroid injections did not experience more pain reduction than the control group; the experimental group also had their knee cartilages deteriorate faster than the control group. While this study was not conducted on spine patients, the significant similarities between the shock-absorbing structures of knee cartilages and spinal discs suggest that the same experiment performed on spine patients would produce similar results.

In addition, there are numerous studies that report that analgesicsor physical therapy used in conventional medicine are not very effective in alleviating pain. Some studies suggest that Eastern acupuncture treatments are more effective than analgesics or physical therapy. In one such study, patients suffering from back pain were randomly divided into two groups. One group was given painkillers or physical therapy, while the other was given acupuncture treatment. The group that received acupuncture reported a greater decrease in pain. Even placebo acupuncture therapy, where the needles do not actually pierce the skin and only sharp stimuli are applied to the surface of the skin, proved more effective than physical therapy or painkillers. The results of this research were published in Pain, the most prestigious journal in pain medicine research.

There is no need to endure pain just because the best course of treatment is often to leave the disc to heal itself. Natural healing can only be effective when the patient is able to carry on with their regular activities without pain interfering. While there are many ways to reduce pain, it is recommended to seek out effective treatments that do not additionally damage the discs, such as acupuncture.

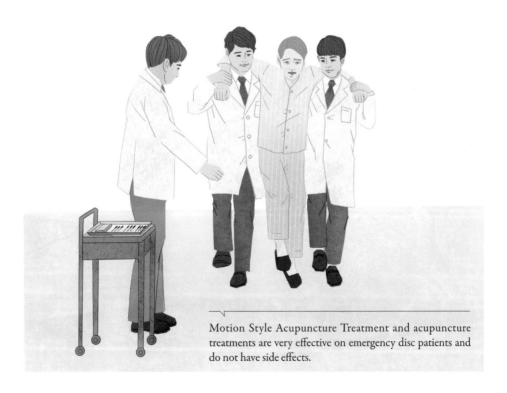

Motion Style Acupuncture Treatment and acupuncture treatments are very effective on emergency disc patients and do not have side effects.

4. Are Re-Operations Necessary for Relapses After Disc Surgery?

Discs Become Weaker with Every Surgery

Tae-min Choi (male, age 45) visited the hospital 4 years ago because of pain in his leg. The hospital examined him and found that there was a problem in the disc between L4 and L5 in the lumbar spine. The doctor recommended surgery.

Wanting to ensure his recovery, Choi asked, "Will surgery really cure my condition? Won't the condition come back?"

"If the operation goes well, the chances of recurrence are less than 5%. You don't have to worry too much," was the doctor's response.

Relieved by the doctor's reassurance, Mr. Choi decided to undergo surgery. For several years after the operation, Mr. Choi encountered no problems and thought the surgery a success. However, three years following his surgery, his back and legs began to hurt again. He was confused because he had thought, just as the doctor had suggested, that the surgery would completely cure him and rid him of his pain.

When Mr. Choi returned to the hospital, the doctor told him that the section that had previously been operated on was fine, but that another disc, between the L5 and L6, had protruded. The doctor recommended he undergo another surgery. Mr. Choi became skeptical because the effects of his last surgery had lasted only 4 years, and decided to visit Jaseng Hospital of

Korean Medicine to seek out Korean medicine treatments.

Many back disc patients receive operations anticipating a complete cure. They believe that removing the protruded discs will not only eliminate the pain, but also restore the discs to full health. This is a devastating mistake. The surgery may make patients feel like they are completely cured by eliminating the associated pain, but in reality, their spine and discs have deteriorated considerably.

In most cases of surgery, the discs that have protruded and are pressing down on the nerves are excised. In order to remove the protruding discs, holes are drilled into the vertebral bones, or parts of the bones are removed. This helps the surgeon visualization and remove the problematic discs. It would be ideal to precisely remove just the protruding discs, but that level of precision is impossible. In the process, the muscles and ligaments surrounding the discs are disrupted as well.

Of course, the wounds will heal with time. There is no guarantee that all of the structures will fully recover. Also, if the compromised muscles or ligaments do not heal properly, they will not be able to provide rigidity to the discs, increasing the risks that the discs will herniate or rupture again.

Furthermore, if the bony structures of the spine are removed, this may compromise the structure of the spine as well.

When the discs are protruding, this indicates that they are no longer able to function properly. Incising the protruded discs weakens them, making it necessary for the surrounding muscles and ligaments to compensate for this weakness. However, because the surgery has weakened the muscles and the ligaments, the condition of the discs with inevitably worsen.

As explained, surgery cannot fundamentally treat herniated discs but ends up weakening the discs. What will happen if another surgery is conducted when the disc herniation recurs? The surgeon will have to again remove or incise the vertebral bones, muscles, and ligaments, further weakening the spine and discs.

The prognoses for reoperation are often not favorable either. The chance of success decreases with every reoperation. While the initial surgery has a success rate of 70 – 80%, the second surgery has a much lower success rate of 50%. If a patient undergoes surgery for the third time, the success rate is no higher than 30%. The subsequent lowered chances of success imply that there is a higher chance of recurrence. Since chances of success are lower reoperation and repeated surgery further damages the spine and discs, patients with recurrent disc problems must be extra cautious when considering their treatment options.

"Procedures" Are Also Surgeries

Some patients say, "When I said that I didn't want more operations, the hospital recommended a 'procedure.' They said that it's a non-surgical treatment that is safer and provides faster recovery. Will I get better with this procedure?"

Even conventional medicine hospitals do not automatically recommend surgery these days. Before considering surgery, they conduct non-surgical treatments first. If these interventions are not successful, then surgery is recommended. Non-surgical treatments in conventional medicine include "procedures." Even though these treatments called "procedures" do not make large incisions in the skin, some still utilize a small hole for an endoscope to enter and employ a technology that induces phenomena like high-frequency waves.

Patients may think that since the incision made on the skin is comparatively smaller, they will have quicker recoveries. This is false. Regardless of whether a small hole is made via an endoscope to remove the protruding discs or to separate the nerves sticking to the discs, such invasive "procedures" will likely damage the ligaments and muscles in the process.

Even with minimally invasive radiofrequency procedures, it is difficult to precisely aim the waves at the protruding discs with resulting desiccation. As such, these procedures will distribute the radiofrequency waves to an entire disc, damaging and shrinking the entire discs in an attempt to reduce the pressure of the focal protruding discs. These types of treatments accelerate the degenerative processes of the discs and therefore result in weakening them. Furthermore, due to the decrease visual field of an endoscope the surgeon may damage organs surrounding the discs.

"Procedures" and surgeries are fundamentally the same, with the only difference being the size of the incision. Both types of treatments irreversibly damage the structures surrounding the discs.

Also, there is no evidence whatsoever that "procedures" are safer than surgery. "Procedures" also damage the spine, discs, and surrounding structures, just like surgery, thereby accelerating the degeneration.

Most "procedures" are more similar to surgery than non-surgical treatments. Non-surgical treatments must only refer to treatments that do not irreversibly damage the discs. It is important that patients know the differences between "procedures" and non-surgical treatments.

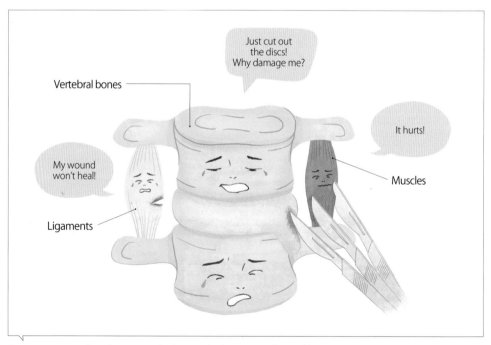

Surgery on protruding discs can easily damage the bones, muscles, and ligaments.

Non-Invasive Korean Medicine Treatment Is the Answer

When faced with a recurrent herniated disc, non-invasive treatments are recommended in place of other operations. This is because discs that have been weakened through surgery will worsen further if they are operated on again.

Conventional medicine and Korean medicine have different approaches to non-invasive treatments. Non-invasive treatments in conventional medicine include physical therapy, pharmachologics, injection treatment, and "procedures," while non-invasive treatments in Korean medicine focus on acupuncture, herbal medicine, pharmacopuncture, and Chuna manual therapy. Since no surgeries are conducted in Korean medicine, all treatments offered in the discipline are non-invasive.

Korean medicine treatments do not irreversibly damage the discs, and they are highly effective. From 2011 to 2014, Jaseng Hospital of Korean Medicine recruited 120 patients suffering from failed back surgery syndrome and provided them with 16 weeks of integrative Korean medicine treatments (including herbal medicine, acupuncture, electroacupuncture, pharmacopuncture, and Chuna manual therapy) to study their effects.

The recruited patients were those who had complained of persisting pain even after spinal surgery or those whose symptoms had returned within 1 year of surgery. They often suffered from severe back pain or lower extremity pain in daily life.

The degree of pain was measured using the visual analog scale (VAS) system. In this method, patients indicated their pain levels on a visual analog scale, with 0 indicating no pain, and 10 indicating highly intense pain. When the study first began, patients reported a pain of level 6 or higher. After the treatments were complete, the majority of the subjects reported lower pain scores on the VAS, indicating that their back and lower extremity pains had been alleviated. Eighty patients (66.7%) reported that their pain levels had reduced by more than 50%. In the follow-up study conducted 1 year later, 80% of the subjects reported that their pain and function had improved.

These treatment results are quite notable. Patients who suffer from failed back surgery syndrome are those whose pain persists after surgery, indicating that they suffer from chronic back pain. As reported in many other studies, only 10% of such patients experience improvement in pain levels after undergoing integrative conventional medicine treatments that combine analgesics, injections, and physical therapy. They may also undergo a separate surgery that permanently implants a stimulation device meant to alleviate pain by electrically stimulating the spinal cord. Even this procedure is considered successful with only a 50%reduction in pain. The results of this research were published in Plos One, a peer-reviewed open access published by the U.S. Public Library of Science.

Conventional medicine and Korean medicine not only have differing treatment effects but also different goals of treatment. Conventional medicine focuses on treating the resulting symptoms, rather than the causes of those symptoms. For disc herniation treatment, this means administrating anti-inflammatory drugs to handle inflamed nerves that are irritated by protruded discs, as well as removing the discs. Because only the symptoms are treated and the underlying causes of the condition are left unaddressed, the discs can always relapse into a ruptured or herniated state.

On the other hand, Korean medicine aims to treat the root causes; Why do discs herniate? Do discs pop out suddenly or spontaneously? The answer to these questions is "No." When people maintain bad postures, abnormal amounts of pressure are applied to the discs. Also, the muscles and ligaments in the back that support the back gradually atrophy, worsening the disc herniation condition. Although it is important to reduce the pain associated with herniated discs, it is crucial to resolve the underlying causes of the condition.

Acupuncture is used in Korean medicine for its strong analgesic effect, providing patients with the ability to endure the condition without undergoing surgery or procedures. Because discs are naturally healed over time, it is very important to reduce pain to help patients endure any painful symptoms until their bodies can heal themselves.

Although herbal medicine can provide analgesic and anti-inflammatory effects, its fundamental functions are to stimulate the recovery of damaged nerves on and around the protruding discs, in addition to strengthening the muscles and ligaments in the vicinity. Chuna manual therapy is a form of treatment that corrects distorted vertebral bones to reduce the amount of pressure applied to the discs. Furthermore, it helps patients correct their postures, thereby reducing the chances that their back pain will return. Pharmacopuncture is a form of treatment that uses herbal medicine to stimulate nerve and disc recovery through acupoints.

Although they are slightly different, Korean medicine treatments all seek to eliminate the root causes of disc conditions. Since treatments are effective in eliminating the causes, the chances of recurrence are significantly reduced. Patients suffering from recurring symptoms need Korean medicine treatments even more. This is because recurrence can only be prevented when the underlying causes are addressed without further damaging the discs.

5. Does All Back Pain Indicate Herniated Discs?

There Are Many Causes of Back Pain

Many patients suspect a herniated discs when they first experience back pain. However, various factors can cause back pain, and damage to the discs is only one of the many possibilities. Pain can be caused by ruptured discs and a leaking nucleus pulposus that compress the nerves, or by lesions on the discs themselves. On the other hand, patients may suffer from back pain when the discs are not damaged at all, and the surrounding muscles or ligaments are instead damaged.

In fact, discs and surrounding muscles and ligaments complement each other. Even if someone is born with discs that are congenitally weaker, if their muscles and ligaments are able to support the discs, there will be a low risk of disc rupture. In general, discs are weakened because of the heavy load they bear. If the surrounding muscles and ligaments are damaged, or are too weak to provide support, the discs will easily rupture.

In the end, both damage to the discs themselves and damage to the surrounding muscles and ligaments can induce disc pain.

Even with the same kinds of back pain, different patients will have varying causes, which must be accurately identified to effectively treat the pain. If the pain is caused by the nucleus pulposus leaking out of the ruptured discs compressing the nerves, the nucleus pulposus must be absorbed back into the body, so that it no longer compresses the nerves. If the surrounding muscles and ligaments are the problem, the damaged supporting organs must be treated and strengthened.

There may be other reasons for back pain other than discs and their supporting muscles and ligaments. In such cases, the symptoms will be similar to those of disc herniation, but treating the discs will not alleviate the pain. If the discs are the root cause, then disc treatments should resolve the pain. However, if such treatments do not improve the symptoms, this serves as an indication that the source of pain is elsewhere.

In fact, many patients mistake their back pain for symptoms of disc herniation. A disc herniation cannot automatically be considered the cause of low back pain; many different possibilities must be explored to identify the true conditions behind the symptoms. That way, appropriate treatment can be employed.

Guillain-Barré Syndrome Has Symptoms Resembling Herniated Disc

"My back and calves hurt as if they are about to burst. The symptoms worsen when I am walking," said a woman in her mid-50s visiting the hospital, as she complained about pain in her back and legs. She reported that the simultaneous pains in the back and legs began appearing about one week after she had suffered from a nasty cold.

The symptoms only worsened as she waited for the pain to subside, so she had visited another hospital about 20 days prior to visiting Jaseng to receive MRI scans. As a result, she was diagnosed with a lumbar disc herniation, and the doctor recommended surgery. But because the patient did not want surgery, she visited Jaseng Hospital of Korean Medicine.

The MRI image itself was sufficient to suspect a herniated disc. To find out why she could not stand, we conducted a deep tendon reflex test. Deep tendon reflex is a phenomenon in which the muscles in the knees, elbows, and achilles tendons contract when these tendons are struck. The patient's reflexes were absent. Her Babinski sign was normal. Babinski sign is a reflex in which the big toe extends when the foot is scratched from the heel towards the big toe along the outer edge of the foot. The reflex is seen when there are injuries of the brain and/or the spinal cord. There were no other neurological signs or symptoms such as appetite, digestion, headache, and pupillary reflexes. Although her muscle strength was weaker than normal, she was able to ambulate because the muscles were strong enough to walk. We determined that the inability to weight bear was due to the pain.

We admitted her for inpatient care after determining her to be a typical spine patient. We provided herbal medicine, acupuncture, and physical therapy. On the second day, however, the patient suffered from a sudden paralysis of her lower extremities that rendered her non-ambulatory. She was also not able to move voluntarily. She also complained that both her feet were numb and her finger tips were cold.

On the third day, her lower extremity paresis worsened. As time passed, her upper extremity strength decreased as well, and the neck pain persisted.

To determine whether there were cervical disc issues and cervical myelopathy, we conducted an MRI scan on the cervical spine. Although there were the expected abnormalities on the MRI images, we considered other diseases that could cause weakness in the upper and lower extremities. Considering her history of progressive paralysis, loss of deep tendon reflexes, and upper respiratory tract infections, we suspected Guillain-Barré syndrome.

Guillain-Barré syndrome is an acute paralytic disease in which the peripheral nerves are inflamed, causing the insulating material called the myelin sheath that surrounds the axons (the branch that extends from the body of the nerve cells) to peel off. As in the case of this patient, it is known to be an autoimmune disease that suddenly occurs within about 10 days after suffering from mild fevers, upper respiratory tract infection, or non-specific virus infections.

When suffering from this disease, patients cannot place weight on their lower extremities, and the symptom spreads to the upper limbs, causing loss of muscle strength. This is called symmetric ascending motor paralysis. Other than that, minor sensory abnormalities such as the degradation or loss of deep tendon reflex are observed. Some patients experience autonomic ataxia accompanied by difficulty breathing and changes to blood pressure and pulse fluctuations.

Diseases that have symptoms similar to those of Guillain-Barré syndrome include cervical myelopathy caused by disc herniation. Myelopathy is a disease in which discs rupture to press down on the spinal cord causing irreversible damage to it. This disease has symptoms similar to those of Guillain-Barré syndrome, such as numbness and paraesthesia in the limbs, feelings of weakness, reduced lower limb strength, and difficulty with ambulation due to discomfort.

Because this patient had similar symptoms, it was easy to mistake Guillain-Barré syndrome as simple back pain due to disc herniation. Because she was older, the MRI images were more likely to show signs of disc degeneration, and she had also suffered from back and leg pain before visiting the hospital. Moreover, because Guillain-Barré syndrome manifests unclear symptoms at its early stages, it was not easy to make an accurate diagnosis.

There are, however, clear differences in symptoms. Herniated disc patients experience loss of strength in certain muscles controlled by certain nerves. For example, when the nerves that connect to the right leg are compressed the right leg will experience numbness and pain. On the other hand, Guillain-Barré syndrome is characterized by l bilateral leg weakness and pain, rather than the symptoms being isolated in certain muscles.

What would have happened if this patient hurriedly decided to undergo surgery just because her MRI scan images showed signs of lumbar disc herniation? It was fortunate that the patient delayed her surgery and turned to other medical professionals that carefully observed the progress of her condition, leading them to diagnose the real disease process.

As demonstrated by this case, common low back symptoms must be observed closely to distinguish them from those of other, lesser-known diseases. Because the misdiagnosis in this case with recommendation to have surgery, it was published in an international academic journal, providing valuable lessons for many medical professionals.

Piriformis Syndrome and Arteriosclerosis Are Other Causes of Back Pain

There is one common disease not caused by disc abnormalities that have symptoms similar to those of lumbar disc herniation. It is piriformis syndrome. The piriformis muscle attaches to the femur from the sacrum (tailbone), and part of a group of six muscles that help move the femur. The sciatic nerve, which is responsible for motor control and sensations of the legs, pass either below or straight through this muscle. When the piriform muscles compress the sciatic nerves, pain and possibly numbness in the hip, back of the thighs, and sometimes the calves and feet. This is called piriformis syndrome.

Broadly speaking, piriformis syndrome is a type of pelvic neuralgia that develops when the piriform muscles become abnormally thick, inflamed, or intensely contracted and compresses the sciatic nerves. It can also develop when there is an injury to the pelvis or the buttocks. This disease causes pain in the buttocks and posterior thighs. In some cases, the pain can radiate to the posterior thighs, legs, and calves and misdiagnosed as a lumbar disc herniation.

Piriformis syndrome is quite common. A significant portion of patients who successfully undergo lumbar disc surgery but experience continued leg numbness and pain are in fact suffering from piriformis syndrome. Unless the piriform muscles in the pelvic region are constantly relaxed and then strengthened through rehabilitation exercises, the symptoms will persist. No amount of treatment on the lumbar discs will relieve the symptoms until the causes of the condition are addressed. The most frightening thing is that the symptoms of the syndrome can recur frequently, making patients and doctors believe that disc herniation has recurred, and thus leading them to another spinal surgery.

Circulatory disorders such as arteriosclerosis can also cause back pain. When examining patients, doctors often come encounter patients whose arteries have been blocked to cause pain in their back and legs. The tissues and nerves in our bodies can only maintain their functions when sufficient oxygen and nutrients are being supplied to them. When blood vessels are blocked, not enough oxygen reaches certain tissues, degrading their functions and causing pain.

In most cases, blockages in the blood vessels occur in the inguinal (groin) region or legs. In such cases, the symptoms are similar to those of spinal stenosis. The temperatures of the two feet differ significantly, and the symptoms worsen in the winter. It is easy to observe the lack of activity of the blood by palpatine the groin region or the back of the foot. An accurate diagnosis can be reached by testing, but such indirect methods can also be used to tentatively diagnose whether there is arteriosclerosis.

Due to the Westernization of eating habits in Koreans, people are consuming more high-calorie and high-fat foods, and more people are being diagnosed with arteriosclerosis. Caution must be exercised, since there are more cases of back or leg pain caused by circulatory diseases, such as arteriosclerosis, than might be expected.

Some back pain and leg pain are caused by diabetes and peripheral neuritis. Peripheral neuritis is a condition in which the functions of peripheral nerves in the hands and feet are damaged due to excessive alcohol consumption or prolonged diabetes. When the causes of back pain are diabetes or peripheral neuritis,the leg pain is more severe than the back pain. Many patients that fall into this category complain that both their legs feel numb and painful, as opposed to just one side of their back or just one leg, as in the case of back disc herniation.

As shown, not all back pain indicates a disc herniation. Spinal stenosis, spondylolysis, and other spinal diseases, as well as other disease processes, have symptoms that are similar to those of disc herniation. Back pain caused by such other diseases requires the doctor to patiently and carefully diagnose the condition based on extensive or outside knowledge. This process is necessary because the pain will not go away unless the correct causes and conditions contributing to back pain are found and treated.

6. Should Pain Treatment Be Prioritized?

Pain Treatment Is Not Everything

Most disc herniation patients present to the hospital when they feel pain. Some patients visit the doctor complaining about extreme pain caused by sudden disc ruptures, but more patients present after suffering from pain for quite some time.

Since they are visiting the hospital for pain, their only concern is pain alleviation. They seek a quick of their pain, regardless of the method. The same goes for medical professionals as well. They seek to alleviate the pain prior to beginning the actual treatment. It does not make sense to tell the patient to ignore the pain and then proceed to treat other aspects of the disease.

The problem, however, is the next stage of the disease. Many patients decide for themselves that their disc conditions have resolved when their pain subsides, and declare that they do not need treatment anymore. This is a dangerous conclusion.

Since disc herniation does not develop overnight and gradually develops over time, it takes time to cure the condition. Visiting the hospital to receive one or two sessions of treatment can quickly reduce pain, but the underlying causes will not have been addressed. Feeling safe in the absence of pain when the root causes remain is dangerous, as disc herniation will only worsen without treatment.

A male patient in his mid-30s visited the hospital,with complaints of back pain. MRI scanning indicated that his discs had not ruptured, which explained the fact that his pain that was less severe. However, the situation was dire. There were 4 discs that were dark black, indicating disc degeneration. Normal discs, which hold in a significant amount of moisture that makes them soft, appear white in MRI images. When discs appear black, this indicates that have dehydrated and thus causing degradation. This, in turn, means that the discs cannot absorb shock properly. Discs must be able to reduce friction and shock between the vertebral bones when the human body is active. Degraded discs, however, cannot properly absorb such shock, contributing to the weakening of the back and worsening of the pain. It was only a matter of time before the patient's discs protruded even further.

Because the discs had not protruded enough to press down on the nerves, the pain subsided easily after 2 to 3 sessions of treatment, the pain disappeared, and the patient no longer required treatment. However, as shown in the MRI images, the patient's situation was worse than that of other patients who had only one protruding disc. Since the discs had hardened and were unable to absorb shock, there was significant risk that the

Normal MRI image

MRI image with 4 degraded discs

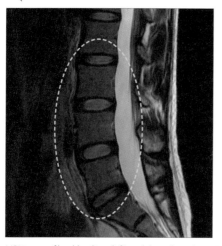 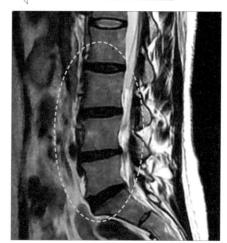

MRI image of healthy discs (left) and that of a male patient in his 30s with 4 black degraded discs (right)

disc extrusion would progress even more quickly. Giving up further treatment meant that he would have to live with four time-bombs that could blow up at any given minute.

The patient was an office worker who frequently worked overtime and consumed a lot of alcohol. He also said that he smoked as much as a pack a day when he was stressed. His lifestyle was filled with bad habits that contributed to back disc herniation.

Since he sat down for most of his day, except for when he was sleeping, there must have been significant stress on his back. Since he did not move very much and smoked, his body's blood circulation would have been restricted more than recommended, preventing the discs from receiving the required amounts of oxygen and nutrients. As a result, this man in his 30's had discs that were degraded as much as those of people in their 50's.

What would have happened if the patient continued his previous lifestyle just because the pain subsided, ignoring all the potential dangers? The degeneration process may have accelerated, and he may have been carried into the hospital on a stretcher one day with severe pain.

Pain treatment is not the entire disc treatment process. It is only the beginning. If patients do not wish to experience more pain from progressed disc herniation, they must continue treating their condition even after the pain subsides. They must try to figure out the underlying causes behind disc herniation, and work to eliminate those causes. If bad life habits are the problem, the habits should be corrected, and if weak muscles and ligaments are the issues, the patients should engage in more exercise to strengthen their muscles and ligaments. These are the ways to prevent further progression or recurrence of disc herniation.

More Important in Old Age

There are patients in their teens and 20s who suffer from herniated discs. Mr. Kim was such a patient. Mr. Kim suffered from ruptured discs at the age of 16 during intense exercise. He underwent surgery for his ruptured discs. Although his discs had ruptured, he had a healthy spine, as well as strong muscles and ligaments. As such, his doctor was confident that the surgery would cure him. The disc symptoms returned after several years, however, and Mr. Kim visited the hospital, where the doctors recommended another operation. Because he did not want another surgery, Mr. Kim decided to visit Jaseng.

I am torn when I come across young patients who suffer from back pain like Mr. Kim. Assuming that our average life expectancy is 80 years old, Mr. Kim will have to live with a poor back for about 60 more years. Of course, with proper management, he will be able to maintain a healthy back for at least 60 years. However, the management process would have been much easier if he did not undergo surgery when the discs first ruptured. Because he was young, non-invasive treatments would have healed his discs. But the surgery bore holes into his vertebral bones and the surgical knife severed his muscles and ligaments. I was even more saddened because the damage from the surgery could not be reversed.

More important than adequate treatment for disc herniation is continued maintenance of health. This is especially true for chronic back disc patients. Compared to acute back disc patients, chronic back disc patients are less sensitive to pain. Because it is usually their first time experiencing such pain, acute disc herniation patients tend to react sensitively. On the other hand, chronic back disc patients become more accustomed to the pain over time despite more serious symptoms. Also, due to the distribution of pain, the patient may not think that he or she is experiencing much pain. After such responses, chronic back disc patients often reach a dire situation that cannot be easily treated.

Regardless if the condition is acute or chronic, disc herniation is a sign that the patient's back must be vigilantly managed. Disc herniation is a type of degenerative disease. Even healthy people will experience aging of their discs as they grow older, and as the surrounding ligaments and muscles age, their back begins to suffer more pain. As such, even if one is not a disc patient at the moment, he or she needs to actively manage his or her back condition to maintain a healthy back for as long as possible.

Any back pain has a significant impact on the quality of life. Even if a person lives for 100 years, not being able to walk, sit down, and stand up due to back pain will make life miserable. Such pain may not have mattered as much when the average lifespan was only about 50 to 60 years. If we assume that someone will live for 80 years, a disc herniation that occurs at age 50 means that the person will have to live with back pain for 30 years. That is not an ideal situation. The impending era of longevity can only be enjoyed fully when people make efforts to receive timely treatments and manage their conditions to prevent the recurrence of diseases.

Exercising routinely and maintaining a healthy weight to reduce the stress on the back are also important, but another good practice is to receive regular medical examinations.

In particular, chronic back disc herniation patients are advised to take MRI scans once every 3 to 5 years, even if there is no pain. This kind of management may be neglected if there is little to no pain, but regular health checkups will generate more alertness concerning the condition and encourage healthier practices.

Discs can only be as healthy as the amount of effort made to maintain their good conditions. As the best treatment is prevention, all individuals, whether suffering from disc herniation or not, are strongly advised to take good care of their discs so that they can live happily in this era of increased longevity.

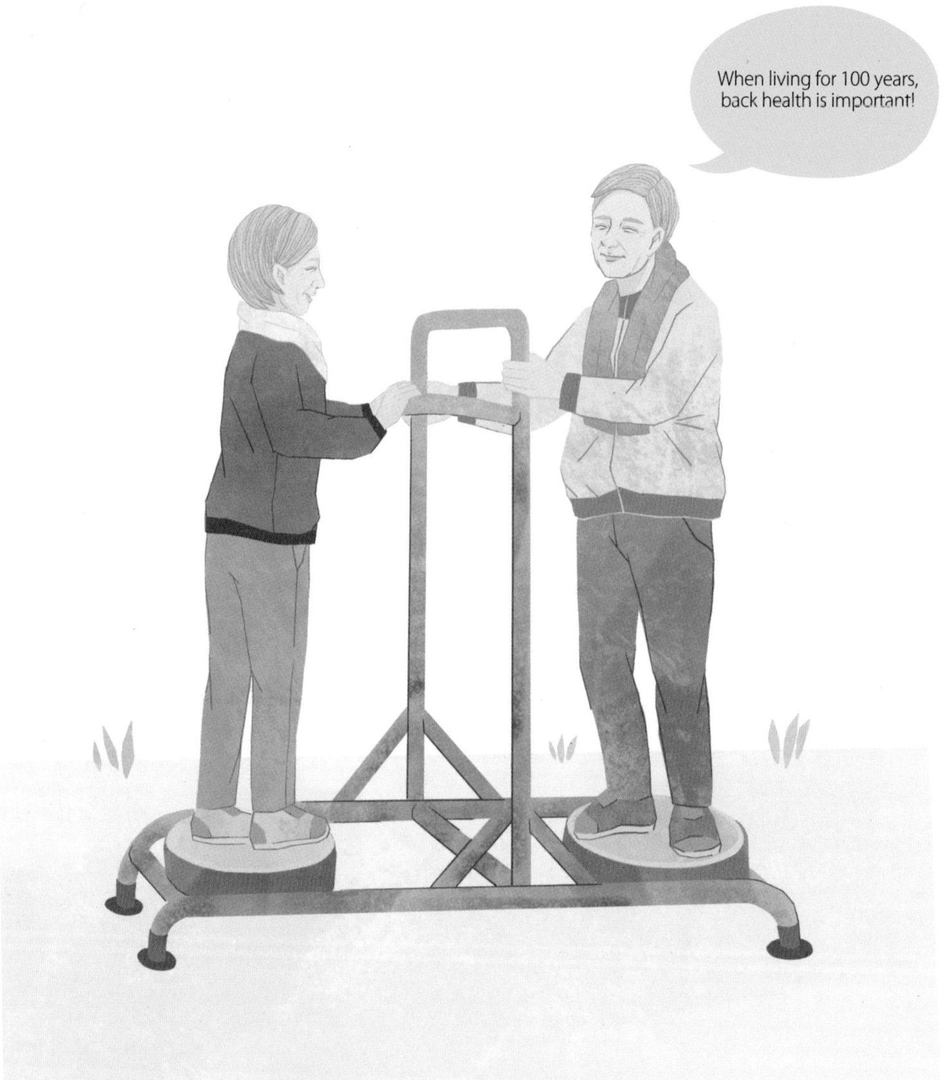
When living for 100 years, back health is important!

7. Is Disc Herniation an Internal Disease?

Disc Herniation Is Also an Internal Disease

"It's a bit embarrassing to say it, but I am a typical upper-middle-class housewife. I've never cleaned my house myself, and I got help when raising my kids. I gained much weight because of increased appetite after childbirth, but I never strained my back... Why do I have disc herniation?" A middle-aged lady who visited Jaseng Hospital of Korean Medicine asked this, saying that she did not understand why she had disc herniation. One of the first things that patients do after being diagnosed for disc herniation is to reflect on their posture and past back use to track down the causes of the condition on their own.

Many people believe that back disc herniation is caused by bad habits or excessive use of the back that can put stress on certain body parts. That is why this patient was also confused about the diagnosis, as she had never physically strained her back before. Even the medical community focuses on abnormalities in the musculoskeletal system when looking at such cases because disc herniation is classified as a musculoskeletal disorder.

Disc herniation, however, can also have internal causes. This patient may have been experiencing arteriosclerosis because she enjoyed high-fat foods and was not very physically active. Arteriosclerosis is an important factor that can cause back disc herniation. Many studies report that the condition is related to arteriosclerosis. Kauppila's research is one such study.

L.I. Kauppila studied how blood supply to the back affects back pain. Cadavers with almost complete loss of function or confirmed to have dysfunctional back arteries and capillaries between ages 16 and 80 were autopsied. The results showed that 88% of them suffered back pain. Among those in the same age range that had normal spinal vasculature, only 22% suffered from back pain. This indicates that those whose spinal arteries were blocked or lost suffered from more severe back pain than those who had healthier back arteries.

Cardiovascular diseases, including arteriosclerosis, are internal factors that can cause disc herniation. In 2015, Jaseng Spine and Joint Research Institute analyzed chronic back pain patients using the data of 23,632 Koreans who participated in the 4th National Health and Nutrition Survey. Among the entire population, 16.6% were shown to suffer from chronic back pain, but among those who had suffered a cardiovascular disease, the prevalence of chronic back pain was twice as high, at 36.6%.

There are many other internal factors that directly or indirectly cause disc herniation. As such, the causes of disc herniation must not be limited to problems in the musculoskeletal system; rather, problems in the internal system must also be considered to enable effective treatment of underlying causes.

If internal factors such as the blood vessels have led to disc herniation, it is very important to foster healthy eating habits. In the past, high-protein foods such as horse bones and shin bone soup were recommended to supplement collagen and other nutrients that strengthen the bones. However, the situation is different today. If modern people with sufficient nutrition sustain excessive consumption of high-protein foods, they can develop cardiovascular diseases, such as arteriosclerosis, caused by elevated cholesterol. As such, patients are advised to refrain from high-fat and high-calorie meals that can increase blood cholesterol levels and cause cardiovascular diseases, and are instead encouraged to consume more fruits and vegetables.

How Do Discs Receive Nutrients?

Just as people need to eat to survive, discs need supplies of nutrition to maintain their health and recover themselves in case of damage. Organs in the human body receive the necessary nutrients and excrete waste products through blood vessels. However, blood vessels are not connected to discs. How, then, do they receive the necessary nutrients? Understanding this process can also shed some light on how disc herniation can have internal root causes. First, it is necessary to closely examine the structure of discs.

Discs are composed of the soft, gel-type nucleus pulposus that is surrounded by the annulus fibrosus. Despite being liquid, the shock-absorbing nucleus pulposus can maintain a certain shape because of the annulus fibrosus and the cartilage endplates located above and below the discs. If we compare discs to a water balloon, the water inside the balloon is the nucleus pulposus, while the rubber balloon skin containing the water is the annulus fibrosus and cartilage endplates.

While discs are not directly connected to blood vessels, some parts of the external annulus fibrosus and cartilage endplates have them. As such, our bodies use the capil-

Structure of disc and nutritional supply to the disc

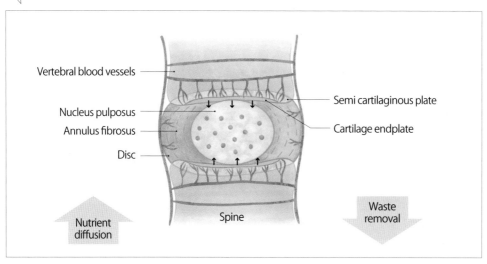

laries that branch out from the back arteries to supply blood to the cartilage endplates. The diffusion caused by the different pressure levels between the cartilage endplates and the disc pushes the nutrients into the discs.

As such, discs receive nutrients through a process that is more complex than is observed in other body parts. When fat accumulates in the back arteries to make them narrower and stiffer through arteriosclerosis, this delicate nutritional supply process becomes even more difficult than it already is.

8. Are Herniated Discs Caused by Bad Posture?

Posture Is No the Definitive Cause

All patients who are diagnosed with disc herniation at Jaseng Hospital of Korean Medicine ask about the cause of their disease: "Why did I develop disc herniation?" "Do discs herniate with bad posture?"

It is natural that patients are curious about the cause of their disease, but it is not easy to point to a single cause that contributed to their conditions. This is because disc herniation often occurs as a result of various combinations of factors.

One of the most common factors discussed is posture. The commonly cited theory is that bad posture places stress on the back. When pressure is constantly applied in everyday life over the course of long periods of time, back discs may rupture eventually. In fact, even until 10 years ago, bad life habits involving bad postures were considered to be the main cause of back disc herniation.

In more recent years, however, the prevalent opinion is that bad posture is not the decisive cause of the disease. Even among office workers who sit in a chair for up to 10 hours a day, some suffer from ruptured discs, while others seem immune to the condition. It is not true that people who do not move or exercise much and prefer to stay in fixed positions develop disc herniation at higher rates. On the other hand, some people who maintain good postures and exercise rigorously in order to prevent disc herniation actually end up suffering from the disease.

As such, there are too many individual cases to generalize that posture is the decisive factor that causes disc herniation. While it is true that posture has an impact on disc herniation, obsessively focusing on that factor can bring more confusion to the debate. It would be disappointing for a patient to see that his or her disc condition is progressing or is not improving even as the patient has made extensive efforts to maintain good postures. Of course, efforts to maintain healthy life habits are very important. Even if posture is not the decisive factor, it does not mean that people can live however they want. Like how little drops of water that can eventually bore a hole in a rock over time, the back cannot withstand sustained physical stress. Although posture is not the sole contributor to the development of disc herniation, patients are advised to maintain good life habits, as posture definitely has an effect.

Fixed Posture Is More Dangerous Than Bad Posture

The size of discs is different in the morning as compared to the evening because of the different amounts of pressure applied to the spine. As discs are under less pressure when the body is lying down, they are larger when measured in the morning right after one wakes up. On the other hand, the discs are smaller in the evening after an entire day of sitting down.

As shown, the sizes of discs vary according to the amount of pressure. Because discs do not have blood vessels, this process of size fluctuations allows the organs to absorb the necessary nutrients. In order for the discs to become larger and smaller through pressure differences, the human body must not be in a fixed posture. A constantly fixed posture means the same amount of pressure is constantly being applied to the discs, preventing them from absorbing the necessary nutrients.

This is why a fixed posture is worse for discs than a bad posture. Even if one has a bad posture, moving around frequently will help discs receive more nutrients. However, even when one maintains a good posture, maintaining such a fixed position for extended periods of time will prevent discs from receiving nutrients, and will possibly weaken them in the process.

There is no one good posture and no one bad posture for discs. Any posture can be bad for discs if it stays fixed for a long time. As such, the best posture for the back is one that changes frequently. The same goes for even the best of postures. Lying down puts less pressure on the spine, making the body feel more comfortable. What would happen, however, when one is always lying down? The lack of change in pressure would affect the discs, reducing the amount of nutrients supplied to the organs. A fixed posture will also stiffen the muscles and ligaments surrounding the discs. Before considering which postures are good, patients will benefit from moving around more frequently and changing postures often.

Does Family History Matter More Than Posture?

Some severe disc patients do not actively seek treatment because of their busy schedules. On the other hand, some patients are excessively worried about their conditions. Such people often have other family members that have suffered from disc herniation.

"My father was not the same person after receiving a lumbar disc herniation surgery, and suffered for almost half his life. I have the same symptoms as my father. What should I do?" This sounds like the patient is overly concerned, but such a concern is not completely unfounded. Although disc herniation is not inherited, family history does play a role in the disease.

One hospital studied 2,500 spinal disease patients for 6 months. 35.8% of the subjects were found to have a family member currently suffering from a back disease. In 23% of the cases, a parent and a child were suffering from a back disease together. This research indicates that having a family member with disc herniation can increase the chance that one also experiences the condition.

Family members often have similar physical constitutions; disc herniation patients often have congenitally weak spinal structures. If a parent has a physical constitution involving a weaker spine, then the child has a greater likelihood of being born with a weaker spine.

Furthermore, family members also share similar life habits. Living together will converge various aspects of people's lives, which means that family members will likely share bad habits that put stress on their back, ultimately increasing the risks of disc herniation. In addition to the congenitally weak spine, the similarities in unhealthy life habits will naturally increase one's chances of developing disc herniation.

Family history, however, should not concern people. Even if they are born with a weaker spine, the back can be strengthened with effort. The risk of disc herniation can be greatly reduced by working to maintain healthy blood vessels that supply sufficient nutrition to the discs, in addition to maintaining healthy life habits.

9. Be Careful About Exercising

Excessive Exercise Can Be Harmful

"I worked out even harder than usual because of my back pain. But it made my back hurt even more, to the point where I can't move that well. Why is that?" A male patient in his 40s came in, complaining unhappily. He expressed frustration, saying that he had been exercising diligently even though his discs were not in such bad conditions.

To prevent disc herniation and recurrences, exercise is necessary. People who suffer from various back pains such as those with back disc herniation are often those who do not exercise regularly. Some statistics show that 60% of people who work in front of a desk all day and do not work out regularly suffer from back pain.

Because discs do not have blood vessels, they cannot circulate fluids and oxygen on their own. As such, frequent walks and movement of the back are the only ways to supply nutrients and oxygen between the bones. However, if one is sitting down for extended amounts of time in a fixed posture, discs suffer from a lack of oxygen, causing them to easily flatten and degenerate. To prevent such degeneration, exercise is absolutely necessary.

Everything, however, should be done in moderation. Excessive exercise can accumulate stress on the spine and surrounding muscles, increasing the toxins.

Walking is an exercise that people can easily do without straining the spine. Simply walking for 30 minutes every day can keep the back healthy. For those who do not have the time to exercise, frequently getting up from the seat and shaking the back can be a great exercise. Shaking the back supplies sufficient oxygen to the discs and surrounding ligaments and other soft tissues, and facilitates blood circulation. This in turn prevents disc herniation. After sitting for 50 minutes, always stand up to walk around or lightly shake the back for about 5 minutes. Gently shaking the back rhythmically will not only alleviate the discs but also reduce the stress on your mind and body.

Exercising in water is also effective. Walking in water is a good exercise that not only strengthens the spinal structure but also builds endurance. In a pool where water comes up to the chest, begin by slowly walking back and forth along a 25-meter lane. Once this feels comfortable, hold the elbow with the hand on the opposite side across the back and walk back and forth. Adjust the intensity of the exercise by gradually increasing speed until you can walk 50 meters.

Swimming is an effective form of exercise for middle-aged people, as the water's buffer and buoyancy relieve the stress on the back, thereby preventing the chance of damage to the joints. Backstroke and crawl are recommended swimming techniques. Because backstroke is the most comfortable and physically balanced style, it is very effective in relieving back pain. A good amount of swimming is 2 or 3 times a week, 30 minutes each time.

However, one should avoid swimming in cold water below 21℃, as doing so can contract the muscles.

Many types of exercise are beneficial for spinal health. The most important thing is to select an exercise that is right for the individual. If it is difficult to choose an exercise or determine the intensity, we recommend consulting a spine doctor to find the right exercise.

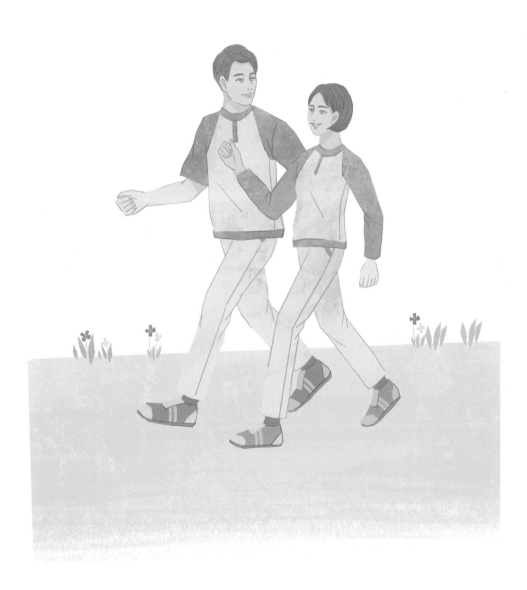

Do Not Exercise When There Is Back Pain

While lack of exercise is a problem for disc patients, excessive exercise with the goal of quicker recovery is an even greater problem. Some patients with strong motivation exercise even harder, enduring their pain or claiming that they cannot feel pain when they work out.

However, patients suffering from pain should not exercise. Working out when the level of pain is higher than usual damages the muscles, which may further worsen the state of the damaged discs. Patients are advised to exercise once the pain subsides to a certain level. They should begin by light exercises such as walking and stationary bicycling, and then gradually increase the intensity and time, taking care that they do not experience pain during exercise.

The most important thing to consider is the current state of health at the time of exercise. As for the patient in this case, his discs had been quite damaged, and his bones and ligaments had been degenerated due to his age. Degeneration is a process of finding a stable state. Engaging in excessive stretching or folding movements that were not normally carried out can place critically dangerous pressure on the discs.

Also, all disc patients experience pain in different ways. During the acute phase, the discs that popped out keep stimulating the nerves, causing much pain. As such, patients should find a posture that is the least painful for themselves. In most cases, patients feel the most comfortable when they are lying on their backs, but some people feel comfortable on their stomachs. In one unusual case, there was a patient who slept sitting down, saying that lying down caused a pinching pain in the discs.

As shown, different patients experience pain in different parts of their bodies, which are damaged to different degrees. It is difficult to say that stretching or yoga is always good for disc herniation. Patients must find the optimal exercise method that fits their own conditions. Working out too much during early stages when the discs have not stabilized may worsen the situation. In order to ensure that exercise is more beneficial than it is harmful, patients must consult a specialist to find the right intensity and method.

2

What Causes
Herniated Discs?

1. The Herniated Disc Is an Inevitable Disease

Herniated Discs in Place of Bipedalism

Four-legged organisms do not suffer from back pain. Humans, being bipedal, are the only species to ever exist that suffer from various spinal diseases, including back disc herniation. The spine skeletal structure of four-legged animals is similar to that of humans. The difference is that the spines of four-legged organisms are parallel to the ground, while those of humans are most often perpendicular to the ground.

The load on the spine is different when it is parallel to the ground versus when it is perpendicular to the ground. Since four-legged animals have spines parallel to the ground and support the spines with four legs, there is much less of a load or burden on the spine. It is different for humans, however. Humans have become the dominant species on Earth, thanks to our ability to walk upright. By being able to stand on two feet, humans have gained the freedom to use both hands; by using both hands, we created countless tools and technologies. That was our secret to becoming the world's dominant species despite our relatively weak physical strength.

By conducting tests on undamaged and healthy discs, the researcher proved that different postures change the pressure placed on discs. The study demonstrated that the pressure applied to the discs was lowest when the subjects were lying down on their back, and that it was the highest when the

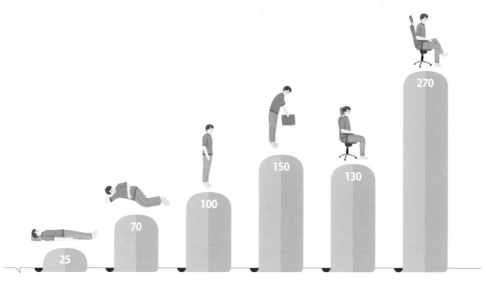

Differences in the pressure on discs depending on the posture. Smaller numbers indicate less pressure on the discs.

subjects were sitting and leaning forward. The weight of disc pressure when standing up straight while crouching forward was higher than simply standing, and both postures placed more burden on the discs than lying down.

Even with the same posture, the pressure placed on discs is higher when crouching or leaning: Crouching while standing applies 1.5 times more force to the discs than when the spine is kept straight; leaning forward with a bent back while sitting applies 2 times more force than when the subject is leaning back. Also, the amount of pressure applied to the discs is 3 times greater when crouching while sitting cross-legged than when simply standing upright.

More burden on the discs leads to weaker discs. Standing straight can alleviate the pressure, but in modern times, people spend much time sitting down. The pressure applied to discs is 1.3 times greater when sitting in a chair than when standing upright. That is why the human spine is put under stress all day long, increasing the chances that disc herniation will occur.

The cervical spine and lumbar spine are especially under heavy pressure.

Since the moment we have been standing on two feet, the spine was doomed to bear the entire body's weight. Fortunately, however, the spine is shaped so that it can bear the weight and withstand external forces.

Broadly speaking, the spine is composed of the cervical, thoracic, lumbar, and sacral-coccygeal vertebra. From a side view, the cervical and lumbar spines are bent slightly backwards and the thoracic spine bends slighty forward, creating an overall "S" shape.

This "S" shape works like a spring. Just as a spring can withstand more weight than a straight object, the "S" shape of the spine distributes the load and lessens the burden on the back. In the end, the "S" shape of the spine is what guarantees the health of the organ.

But just as it often is in life, we lost something when we gained this amazing capability. While having the ability to use both hands, we are now cursed with having to support the entire body's weight with our spine. Except for when we are sleeping, the spine must remain upright all day. This puts an immense load on this body organ.

The weight placed on the spine differs when we are standing up straight and when we are lying down. Nassemson, a pioneer of spinal disc research, studied how the pressure applied to discs changes depending on the posture. He devised a special converter that measures the pressure inside the disc between at L3-4 under various postures and conditions.

However, there is only so much that the "S" shape of the spine can do, even if it distributes the weight load. People who have to stand or sit for extended amounts of time will continuously place significant stress on their back, despite the "S" shape of the spine. This is especially true for the cervical spine and lumbar spine.

The lumbar spine, which supports the lower back, is composed of five vertebrae. The lumbar spine bears 70% of the body weight, a significant portion. As such, these vertebrae are larger than those in the cervical and thoracic spines. The muscles that support the lumbar spine are also quite large. Despite such structures, the lumbar spine is easily

Structure of the Spine

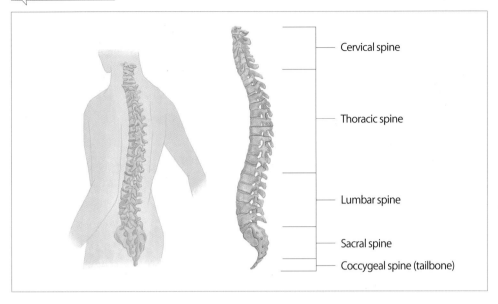

- Cervical spine
- Thoracic spine
- Lumbar spine
- Sacral spine
- Coccygeal spine (tailbone)

damaged because of the heavy weight load and frequent movements. It is, thus not a co-incidence that the lumbar spine is more prone to disc herniation than other parts of the spine. The cervical spine is the section that is second-most prone to disc herniation after the lumbar spine. The cervical spine suffers as much stress as the lumbar spine. Unless the human body is lying down, the cervical spine must support the head, which is of a significant weight. It also moves almost as much as the lumbar spine. As such, cervical disc herniation is as frequent as lumbar disc herniation.

It is natural that disc herniation is more frequent in the cervical and lumbar spines. Even with the best posture, the cervical and lumbar spines will suffer to a certain degree because they are designed to bear the heaviest loads in the human body. One must not, however, think that maintaining good posture is useless. When the human body is designed for the spine to bear so much weight, maintaining bad posture will accelerate the speed at which the spine weakens and degenerates.

If we cannot change the structure of the spine, we must embrace it and learn to cater to it. After that, we can help the spine not suffer any more than absolutely necessary in order to lead happier and healthier lives.

2. Discs Do Not Herniate Overnight

Discs Are Sturdier Than You Think

"I don't know. My discs burst after I sneezed harshly." "My back has never hurt this much until now. But I felt a sharp pain in my back when I was putting my futon back in the closet, and since then, I can't move." Many patients who visit our hospital say something along these lines when doctors ask them about their conditions. What they tell us makes it seem like their discs burst when they were experiencing absolutely no problems before. Discs, however, are not so weak that they burst spontaneously without any preceding reasons.

Of course, discs can rupture when people sneeze or bend their backs to pick up a tissue off the floor. In some cases, back pain can even come after a good night's sleep.

In such instances, it is easy for patients to think that their discs ruptured all of a sudden, but their disc conditions probably had been developing for a long time without them noticing. Like a single drop of water can make a full cup overflow, simply sneezing or bending the back can apply enough shock to rupture already an weakened discs.

In fact, people who claim that their discs suddenly ruptured have blackened discs on their MRI scan images. The coloration indicates that the discs have been weakened as much as possible. While there are individual differences, no one can develop such bad conditions in just a matter of days.

Let's take a look at the structure of our discs. There are 23 discs in our body, between all the vertebrae except for between the cervical levels of C1 and C2. The discs look like mochi rice cakes. A cross-section of the disc reveals that the organ is composed of the gelatinous nucleus pulposus, which is surrounded by the annulus fibrosus, a fibrous structure, on all sides. Eighty percent of the nucleus pulposus is composed of water, and it plays an important role in the disc receiving nutrients and discharging waste.

Without discs, the vertebrae will grind against each other to create friction, delivering unfiltered shocks to the brain. With every movement of the spine, the discs can either shrink while being pressed down on or expand, depending on the direction of movement. For example, bending forwards will flatten the front parts of the discs and widen the back parts. Also, when pressure is applied to the back, the discs in the parts where pressure is greater will become thinner, distributing the force in the opposite direction, thereby reducing it.

The nucleus pulposus in discs is mostly water, which means that they are soft, but the surrounding annulus fibrosus is like tough rubber. In addition, strong ligaments and muscles tightly hold onto the discs on all sides, preventing them from bursting even under significant pressure.

Cross-section of the spine

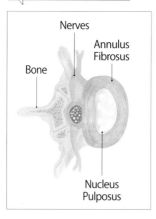

Nerves

Annulus Fibrosus

Bone

Nucleus Pulposus

Cross-section of the disc

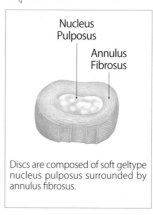

Nucleus Pulposus

Annulus Fibrosus

Discs are composed of soft geltype nucleus pulposus surrounded by annulus fibrosus.

Side view of the disc

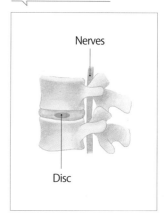

Nerves

Disc

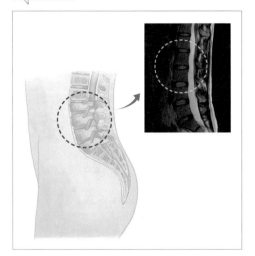

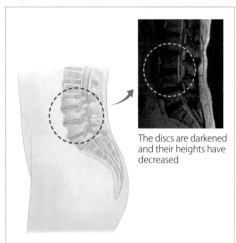

The discs are darkened and their heights have decreased

Small drops of water, however, can bore a hole in rock over time. Even if discs have sturdy structures and are protected by muscles and ligaments, they will gradually weaken under sustained pressure. When the annulus fibrosus that wraps around the nucleus pulposus tears away bit by bit, the disc will slowly begin to leak out and eventually resulting in rupture.

When the disc does not burst, its nucleus pulposus can become harder and darker under sustained pressure. That is why some patients show black discs on MRI scans. The hard and inelastic nucleus pulposus cannot properly help the disc carry out its shock-absorbing function between the vertebral bones.

Disc Herniation Happens in Stages

When discs weaken and cannot withstand pressure any longer, they begin to pop out, bit by bit. When such leaking discs press down on the nerves, they can cause pain. This is what we commonly call herniation of the disc.

Significant amounts of time are required for discs to be able to leak out and press against the nerves. Patients usually do not notice such herniation until the pain starts to bother them. Once discs begin to herniate, it is difficult to bring them back to their original state without extensive efforts. Consistent treatment and maintenance efforts to strengthen the muscles and ligaments, however, can stop the further progression of the disease. But because most patients cannot even undergo treatment when they do not know that their discs are herniating, in most cases, the discs become weaker and end up rupturing.

Disc herniation begins with the water escaping from the nucleus pulposus. A normal, healthy disc appears white on MRI scans, but a disc with less or no water in the nucleus pulposus appears dark. This is a potentially dangerous situation, in which the disc has not ruptured but has lost its elasticity; disc herniation can happen at any moment.

After this state, the annulus fibrosus begins to weaken and tear away. The annulus fibrosus is composed of multiple layers, giving the structure a tough texture. Small tears

Disc extrusion process

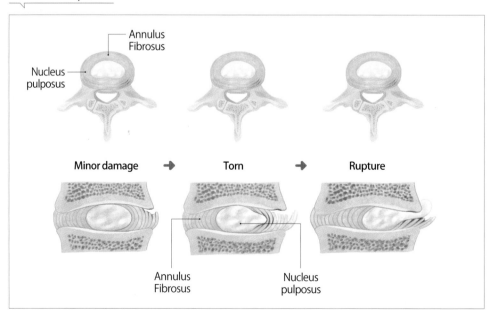

on the annulus fibrosus will not just cause the nucleus pulposus to leak, but in this stage, the disc will begin to herniate in earnest. In such cases, the disc herniates towards the direction where the annulus fibrosus has weakened more. This is called protrusion.

When this progresses further, the annulus fibrosus completely breaks down, causing the nucleus pulposus to leak out and compress the nerves.

Pain ensues when the nucleus pulposus compresses the nerves, and worsens when the nucleus pulposus stimulates the nerves. This late stage is called disc extrusion.

In sum, discs do not burst spontaneously, because disc herniation is a process that takes place gradually. A better way to understand this disease is to think about the risk factors that accumulate over time, and certain events cause the discs to rupture.

3. Why Do Homemakers Suffer More From Herniated Discs?

A Bent Back Leads to More Easily Herniated Discs

It is easy to think that men will damage their discs more frequently than women because the former often engage in more intense physical labor. In reality, however, women suffer from disc herniation more than men do. A higher prevalence of joint diseases also exists amongst women than men. Why is this the case?

In terms of intensity, the types of physical work that men engage in are usually more straining than those of women. However, women, especially homemakers, do work that involves frequent bending and unbending of the spine, even if the individual acts may not be of high intensity. Wiping the floor, washing the dishes, and many other household chores require the worker to bend and unbend the back frequently.

Engaging in such motions will put pressure on the discs and damage them. Even if the damages are small, if they are sustained over long periods, this will cause discs to rupture.

Discs themselves cause the problem in some cases, but in many other cases, the issue is with the facet joints near the discs. Discs absorb shock to lessen the load on the spine bones. They are not the only organs playing this role, however. Discs bear 70% of the total body weight load, while the remaining 30% is borne by the facet joints.

The bending and unbending motions cause only minor damages to the discs, but they will create constant friction in the facet joints and cause them to wear out.

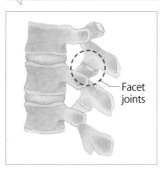

Facet joints near the discs bear 30% of the weight load

Facet joints

Homemakers' knee joints are often quite thick. Engaging in laborious household chores, such as laundry and cleaning, can cause the joints to undergo friction. Osteophytes (needle-like structures at the ends of the bones) are created and grow on the bones to withstand the damage caused by this friction. When such degenerative changes take place in the joints, their functionality significantly decreases, so that the surrounding muscles and organs are forced to take on more stress. The joints thicken in this process.

When the facet joints, which are meant to share the load of the human body with the discs, cannot play their role properly, the patient will begin experiencing disc problems.

This will manifest as back pain. X-ray images alone are not enough to determine whether such pain is caused by discs or facet joints. On the other hand, facet joints can wear out because of problems in the discs. If discs lose moisture and flatten for some reason, the vertebrae above and below the discs, as well as nearby facet joints, will clang against each other to create friction. This makes the vertebral bones and facet joints to wear out faster, which in turn accelerates disc degeneration.

Because women naturally have weaker joints, muscles, and ligaments than men, they suffer more from subluxation. Luxation is the dislocation of the joints; subluxation is the state where the joints are not completely dislocated, but only partially removed diagonally from their normal positions. When the facet joints are subjected to more friction due to the thinning of the discs, subluxation will take place, weakening the spine further. Also, when the facet joints wear out from the friction to degenerate the joints, the joints themselves will become thicker. This narrows the nerve space behind the discs. If discs herniate into this smaller space, the nerves will be compressed more due to the greater pressure, thereby worsening symptoms.

When this condition progresses further, it causes spinal stenosis.

In addition to their weaker bones, joints, muscles, and ligaments, the higher frequency of household chores that involve bending and unbending the back leads to women suffering more than men from disc and facet joint problems. In addition, when they enter menopause, feminine hormone production will decrease, which further weakens their bodies and induces more pain.

Certain Occupations Are More Prone to Herniated Disc

Occupation, as well as sex, is another factor that is closely related to disc health. White-collar workers who are subject to high stress and not much active movement, drivers who are in their seats for extended amounts of time, and farmers and manual workers who use their backs frequently are more prone to disc ruptures than those working in

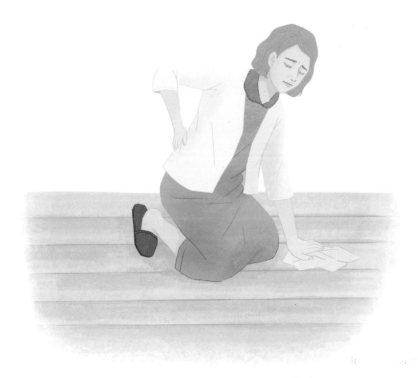

other professions.

Let's take a look at professional drivers. To secure a wider angle of view, most drivers often sit with their backs off the back of their car seats. Also, they are more likely to stay alert to monitor traffic flow, which means that they will be more sensitive and prone to stress. They are at a higher risk of disc herniation because of their postures and the high level of stress that places tension on their backs.

According to one report, more than 60% of professional drivers have received medical care for back pain. Although their job forces them to be sitting down for long hours, drivers are advised to make as much time as possible during their jobs to stretch their tense backs. It is recommended for them to stretch or even lightly exercise outside their vehicles, but if that is not possible, they must move their bodies while sitting down to facilitate blood circulation.

The same goes for white-collar workers. Because office workers are in their chairs for most of their working hours, and because of continued stress and overwork, their muscles are constantly suffering. Many people who work in fixed positions feel that the backs of their necks stiffen, and that their spines are under more stress, causing chronic back pain. Their back pain reduces their work efficiency and has a negative impact on the rest of their lives, which often can lead to clinical depression.

People who work under occupational factors that can burden their backs must take extra efforts to keep their backs healthy. Rather than driving to work, they may benefit from taking public transportation. People who spend many hours of their day sitting down might move more taking public transportation than when driving to work. They should move as much as possible and refrain from overeating or eating too many foods high in calories and fat. Making such efforts can cut the risk of disc herniation in half.

On the other hand, people such as manual laborers and farmers who frequently use their backs should take breaks to rest their backs adequately, and stretch often to relax their tense backs. In particular, workers who need to bend their backs for extended amounts of time will need to make conscious efforts to get up occasionally and stretch their backs.

4. Reasons for Herniated Discs Are Complex

Discs Do Not Herniate for One Reason

"I fell badly during a mountain hike about 10 years ago, and my back started hurting often since then. Didn't my discs rupture because of that incident?" Disc patients often ask if certain situations or events caused their disc herniation.

Of course, patients want to know why their discs have ruptured, but there is not a simple answer. This is because discs do not burst for one single reason.

Of course, a bad fall from 10 years ago may have contributed to the problem.

The shock to the spine suffered from the fall may have weakened the discs, and the patient may have continued to exert excessive force on their back or maintain a bad posture that put stress on the back. Such circumstances may have promoted disc herniation. As explained, physically traumatic events from long ago should be seen as having been a trigger point, rather than a direct cause.

There are so many things that can cause discs to rupture. Since multiple causes work in tandem to rupture discs, it is difficult to judge for certain which factors exactly make discs burst.

In general, however, factors such as family history, bad life habits, and disc degeneration are cited as common causes of disc herniation. These factors indicate that they are not independent, but are highly susceptible to be influenced by each other.

However, the diversity of causes does not mean that prevention is complex or difficult. Since the causes are entangled with each other, the patient's efforts to deal with one specific cause is likely to help resolve other causes as well. For example, a person who is used to a high-calorie and high-fat diet will lessen his or her risk of arteriosclerosis if he or she fixes these bad eating habits.

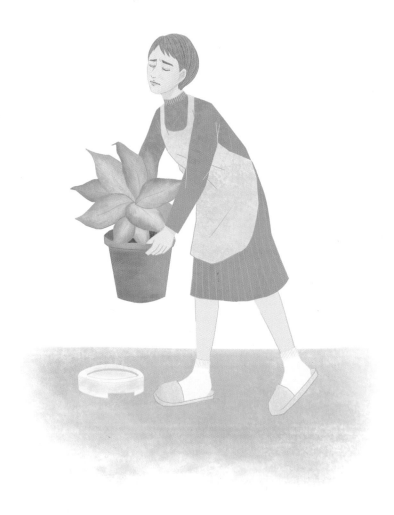

Even patients with family histories of disc herniation may not suffer as much from the condition if they successfully change bad lifestyle habits. As such, rather than obsessing over the causes behind disc herniation, patients are advised to fix what they can among many potential causes.

The same goes for degeneration. Although no one can escape the degenerative effects of aging, the speed of physical degeneration greatly varies from person to person. Some age more quickly, while others boast youthful, healthy backs. The speed of degeneration may differ due to natural genetic factors, but bad habits or diseases can always catalyze degeneration.

The Secret Is the Factor that is Causing Degeneration of Discs

In fact, the spine medicine community focuses more on the causes of spinal degeneration, rather than the causes of disc rupture. Degenerated discs can easily burst when lifting light objects, or even when sneezing lightly.

It is, however, difficult to determine the direct cause of degeneration. Degeneration is generally caused by aging, a natural phenomenon of the human body. It would be nice to explain the degeneration of discs as a natural process of aging, like how wrinkles grow on the skin as one ages, but the reality is much more complicated than that.

In recent years, we have found that disc degeneration affects even teenagers. Since cells are still being generated in teenagers' bodies, it is too early to experience spinal aging during teenage years. However, some teen patients' MRI scan results indicate signs of spinal degeneration that are common for people in their 40s and 50s. Although the average life span is increasing, the degeneration rate of modern people's discs is accelerating.

What are the factors contributing to the degeneration of discs in today's population? There are expected causes. As food has become more abundant and readily available, people have started to consume more high-calorie and high-fat food. In addition, with faster and more convenient transportation methods, people now have much fewer

Research on internal factors of disc herniation

Research characteristics	Results	Author and year of publication
Autopsied 140 bodies ages 16 to 89; patient control study	Patients with blocked or narrowed lumbar arteries experienced more chronic pain than patients without.	Kauppila, 1997
Autopsied 86 male bodies ages 36 to 69; a cross-sectional study	More severe disc degeneration is accompanied by arteries leading to the discs. This is more so for higher lumbar spines. All lumbar disc degeneration is related to lesions in the abdominal aorta.	Kauppila et al., 1994
8,816 male farmers, ages 30 to 49, 13-year follow-up observation	Patients who reported back pain had a higher risk of death due to ischemic heart disease than those who did not.	Penttinen, 1995
606 subjects, Framingham cohort, the average age at 54, 25-year follow-up observation	Abdominal aortic calcification is related to the general disc degeneration.	Kauppila et al., 1997
1,429 women, average age at 71, average 3.7-year follow-up observation	Women with cardiovascular diseases had a higher chance of having back pain and disabilities associated with the condition. Follow-up observations revealed that back pain related disabilities tended to be double in the group with cardiovascular diseases.	Vogt et al., 1997
98,407 women, nurses' health research, ages 30 to 55, 16-year follow-up observation	Disc extrusion, diabetes, hypertension, and high cholesterol were correlated. Subjects who suffered from myocardial infarction prior to age 60 and are currently smoking had a higher risk of disc herniation depending on their daily smoking volume.	Jhawar et al., 2006
902 industrial workers, 27-year follow-up observation	Men with high triglyceride concentration, high diastolic blood pressure, and experience of smoking had a higher chance of suffering from localized back pain. In addition, higher total cholesterol levels, higher triglyceride levels, higher blood pressure, and current smoking habits tended to be correlated to more severe back pain. More risk factors causing cardiovascular diseases were correlated with a higher risk of back pain occurrence.	Leino-Arjas et al., 2006
43 patients, ages 50 to 87, cross-sectional study	The frequency of back pain before surgery was higher than in the group with abdominal arterial obstruction. The back pain of the group with abdominal arterial obstruction was improved after surgery. The study confirmed that treatment of the cardiovascular system can improve back pain.	Shiri et al., 2007
1,484 women, ages 70 to 85, 5-year follow-up observation	Chronic pain was related to mortality caused by heart diseases.	Zhu et al., 2007
8,028, ages 30 to 95, cohort study	Hyperlipidemia and back pain were correlated.	Leino-Arjas et al., 2008

opportunities to move.

The common opinion is that because people spend most of their time sitting down, their backs weaken. Less movement and more food intake increase body weight, increasing the load placed on the back, so that discs age and degenerate more quickly.

While this opinion is quite persuasive, it is difficult to explain everything about disc degeneration in such a straightforward manner. As such, more researchers are studying the causes of disc degeneration with new approaches. Jaseng Hospital of Korean Medicine is also making multifaceted efforts to understand the factors contributing to back disc herniation. While this is not an easy endeavor, we hope to find the fundamental causes of disc herniation to ensure that no one ever has to suffer from ruptured back discs.

5. Do You Need MRI Scans for Herniated Discs?

MRI Is Required to Identify Your Disc Condition

Patients sometimes ask, "Do I need to take the MRI scan?" When patients visit a hospital due to back pain, medical professionals will first take X-ray photos. If they suspect ruptured discs, they move on to conduct MRI scans of the back. Although MRI is the imaging that most accurately displays the physical state of the back, many patients ask the above question because of the relatively high costs.

In fact, there are conflicting opinions regarding how effective MRI scanning can be in diagnosing ruptured discs. A research team took MRI scans of a group of healthy, middle-aged people who had not experienced much back pain and reported that about 30% of them had protruded discs. Since that study, people began to doubt whether MRI scanning is necessary if there is no pain even with ruptured back discs.

This idea that MRI scans are ineffective was supported by the fact that the degree of rupture in the discs does not always correlate to the level of pain.

There has been a study on whether MRI scans enable more effective treatment of disc herniation. A research team based in the U.S. tracked 5,000 back pain patients over the age of 65, categorizing them into patients who took MRI and CT scans since the early stages of their treatment and those who did not undergo any imaging tests. The general effectiveness of treatment in the two groups was the same after one year had passed. The researchers had hypothesized that the group who received imaging tests would have been exposed to customized treatments that would lead to less pain, better treatment effects, and less surgery. However, the results showed no clear differences between the two groups. The results of this study also helped support the idea that MRI scans are not useful.

Despite these studies, however, the spine medicine community collectively believes that MRI scans provide more benefits than losses. Once ruptured, discs cannot be treated quickly. Of course, pain can quickly subside with adequate treatment, but since this does not mean that disc herniation is cured, patients cannot let their guards down. Because discs can continue progressing in the absence of pain, patients must undergo MRI scans to receive proper treatment. MRI scans allow medical professionals to accurately observe the state of the discs and determine the course of treatment that will be most effective.

The results of MRI scans must be sufficiently shared between the medical specialist and the patient. Patient knowledge is important because it allows patients to more proactively participate in the treatment.

Although Jaseng Hospital of Korean Medicine is equipped with X-ray and MRI equipment, many patients bring in imaging test results from different hospitals.

Curiously enough, patients who bring in such images commonly tell us that they have not received a detailed explanation about the state of their discs. They say that their doctor glanced at the MRI images and just told them, "You have disc herniation. It's severe," accompanied by a simple recommendation for surgery or other treatments. The patients say that doctors rarely discuss with them how their disc herniation can progress without intervention, and how they should maintain their discs.

In fact, there are many things to be explained about disc herniation. Patients need to know how disc herniation begins, why their discs look dark on MRI images, and how to ensure that discs receive sufficient nutrition, in addition to much other information related to back health. After taking MRI scans, patients need to hear sufficient explanations about the results from the doctor and appraise their own conditions to be able to consider the right courses of treatment.

Disc herniation patients who have long suffered from diabetes, hypertension, and arthritis have even greater need to take MRI scans. Patients who have been suffering from a chronic disease for extended periods are more likely to have received pharmacological treatment, as well as steroid injections to reduce pain levels. In addition to back treatment, many patients may have received invasive but non-surgical treatments for their shoulders, knees, and other joint conditions. Since their immune systems may have been significantly compromised, older patients must take extra care to identify their disc conditions. In addition to disc conditions, MRI provides detailed images regarding the spinal structure and the state of the surrounding ligaments and muscles. As such, the technology can provide ample information required to treat older disc patients.

You Don't Need MRI Scans for Every Instance of Pain

MRI scanning is a necessary step required to evaluate the state of the discs. It is, however, unnecessary to take MRI scans for every instance of occasional back pain. With a light sprain on the back (torn lumbar ligament), the symptoms will almost disappear with 1 to 2 weeks of treatment regardless of the level of initial pain. If back pain persists even with 2 weeks of appropriate treatment and X-ray images raise suspicions about disc herniation, patients are advised to get MRI scans. In such cases, patients may not have simply sprained their backs; their back discs may have been degenerating for a long time, inducing pain only recently. In particular, if patients who experience frequent and repeated lower back pain have X-ray images of narrow intervertebral spaces, they must have MRI scans to evaluate their precise conditions.

Some patients suffer the grave consequences of not having MRI scans soon enough. The Gangnam branch of Jaseng performs about 500 to 600 MRI scans per month. Among them, there are 2 to 3 rare cases of spine cancer. Such patients who have never experienced symptoms of spine cancer coincidentally discover the disease when they

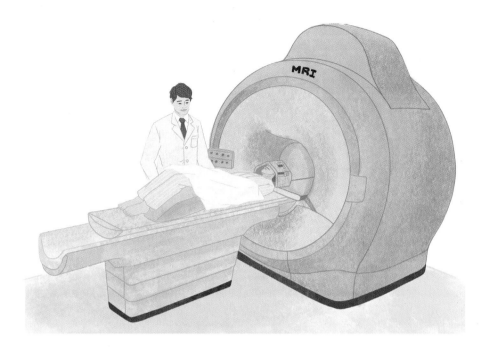

visit the hospital and receive MRI scans to see if they have back disc herniation. In such cases, Jaseng does not engage in disc herniation treatment, and instead refers the patients to university hospitals to undergo spine cancer treatment, thus saving their lives.

In other cases, patients suffer from spinal infections. Among patients who have received indiscriminate injection treatments, those whose immune systems have been compromised can develop back infections. Such back pains caused by infections or tumors are difficult to distinguish from disc herniation if only presented with symptoms. As such, MRI can help in providing the correct diagnosis.

Jaseng Hospital of Korean Medicine provides treatments that integrate conventional and Korean medicine. It employs conventional medical testing such as blood tests, CT, and MRI, whose results are examined and analyzed by conventional medical specialists. Using the information provided, Korean medicine is used to treat the root causes of the disease. The cost of treatment is rather high, of course, because conventional medicine is used for testing and Korean medicine is used for treatment. However, since accurate diagnosis is required for effective treatment, the integration of conventional and Korean medicine is necessary for the health and timely recovery of patients.

Tests for Checking Your Disc Condition

X-Ray Imaging

This is the most basic test used to diagnose spine diseases. Because the bone structure is imaged from many angles, it is easier to observe the structural form of the spine. Diseases such as scoliosis and spondylolysis can be accurately diagnosed with only X-ray images.

Disc herniation, however, is different. While the space between the vertebral bones and the degree of disc degeneration can indicate the possibility of disc herniation, X-ray images are insufficient for identifying the precise location and progression of the potential herniation. This is because X-ray images do not show the discs.

X-ray photo of the cervical spine

MRI image of the cervical spine

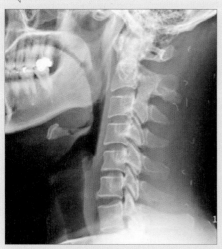 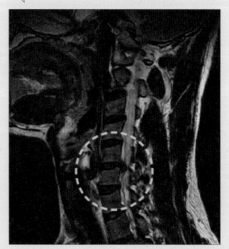

Although the X-ray image (left) does not show whether disc herniation exists, the MRI image (right) can lead to a diagnosis of cervical disc rupture.

Myelogram (Discography)

This testing method complements the weaknesses of X-ray imaging. A contrast medium is injected into the spinal cavity to see the shapes of the discs that have ruptured or "popped out". This method is not used widely since the advent of MRI, but it is still the most effective test for diagnosing internal disc disruption. Since discs do not have blood vessels, they cannot feel pain. If discs are damaged, however, microvessels and nerves can generate and enter into them. Such a change in the structure of the discs causes internal disc disruption. When the contrast medium is injected into the back with internal disc disruption, the patient may feel pain as the needle pierces the discs.

Computer Tomography (CT)

This modality combines X-ray and computer technology. Radiation penetrates the body at a high speed to create cross-sectional images of the internal human body. Because it shows different cross-sections of the vertebral bones that cannot be seen with the plain X-ray, CT can isolate the precise location of disc herniation, as well as the severity of the condition.

Furthermore, it is effective in determining whether the disc surface has calcified, if discs have degenerated, or if spinal stenosis has occurred. Computerized tomography scans are less expensive and quicker to use, but because of the low image resolution for soft tissues such as ligaments, an accurate diagnosis is difficult.

Magnetic Resonance Imaging (MRI)

Magnetic Resonance Imaging is a testing method where the magnetic properties of the substances that make up the human body are measured – the results of which are processed by a computer to create images. Unlike CT scans that can only take cross-sectional photos, MRI images can be taken at different angles. Because the technology uses magnetic fields, it is not harmful to the human body. Magnetic Resonance images also show cartilages, muscles, nerves, surrounding tissues, and vertebral bones, enabling medical professionals to check the protrusion of the discs. However, MRI scanning is relatively expensive and the imaging times are quite lengthy.

Muscle Strength Test for Back Functionality

This testing method uses muscle strength testing devices to determine the current functionality of the patient's back or neck. The method can show abnormalities in the flexion and extension of the back, as well as the current state of muscle strength. It also enables the comparison of muscle strength before and after treatment. In addition, it can be used effectively to prescribe exercise therapy depending on the pain level and symptoms of the patient.

Electromyography Testing the State of the Nerves and Muscles

Electromyography is a useful method that tests all abnormalities within the motor unit to identify the location, degree, progression, and recovery of the diseased area. Weak electrical stimulation flows into the nerves, whose electrical signals are recorded. For disc diseases, electromyography is conducted to investigate symptoms such as tingling sensations in the limbs or weakened muscle strength.

Arteriosclerosis Test Measuring Vascular Age and Circulatory Disorders

Arteriosclerosis test measures the blood flow in the limbs to determine the degree of arteriosclerosis and changes in the thickness of the blood vessels. This test can provide the vascular age – a way of measuring the health of blood vessels in the patient, and identify vascular disorders.

In Korean medicine, arteriosclerosis tests are conducted to preemptively check for circulatory disorders. Because the test can discover and prevent circulatory system diseases early on, it is often used in medical checkups for middle-aged or older patients. It is also used to check for circulatory issues that can easily accompany disc diseases. The arteriosclerosis test is performed with the patient lying down and with measurement tags attached to the limbs. Test times are relatively short and there is no stimulation, making the test more convenient.

Infrared Body Heat Test

The infrared body heat test measures the body temperature to gauge the degree of back disc herniation. It shows areas with high body temperatures in red and those with low body temperatures in blue, indicating abnormalities in the body. When herniated or protruding discs compress the nerves, the neural signals are not easily transmitted. In this case, the body temperature drops and shows up in blue during the infrared test. In contrast, when the affected nerves are inflamed, the body temperature in the area increases, showing up in red during the test. Whether it is red or blue, if the area shows a more extreme contrast than other areas, this indicates a severe back disc herniation.

Even without disc herniation, neurological diseases such as diabetic peripheral neuropathy show up in blue during the test, as in the case of disc herniation. Because the physiological abnormality is shown in colors, it is important for the medical professional to properly identify whether the color differences are caused by disc herniation or by other conditions.

3

From Causes to Cures:
Jaseng's Non-Invasive Treatments

1. Herniated Disc Requires Surgical Intervention: How Was This Preconception Changed?

MRI Disproves "Herniated Disc = Surgery"

A patient said, "I sprained my back several months ago while playing golf, and I couldn't move at all. When I went to the hospital, they told me that my discs burst and that I needed surgery. Back then, I was in no position to undergo surgery and I did not want to. So, I received only Korean medicine treatments. The pain started subsiding with the treatment, and I feel just fine now. I think my disc is completely better."

Until recently, many people did not believe that Korean medicine treatments alone, without surgery, could completely cure disc abnormalities. Most people thought that ruptured discs, even after the pain dissipates still required a surgical intervention at some point.

In fact, as recently as 30 years ago, the general consensus was that surgery was the only option for relieving the pain from disc herniation. Despite the fear and anxiety associated with surgery, most believed there was no other option to treat back pain caused by disc herniation. Patients would endure the pain, delaying surgery until the last moment.

Over time, even after surgery, a significant portion of patients still experienced pain. Patients with disc herniations who believed that surgery would free them from chronic back pain, but did not benefit much from the operation, shared with others that "surgery is useless." These comments caused more people to become reluctant to have suregry, and others shifting toward non-invasive treatments in place of surgery to alleviate their disc conditions.

In the 1980s, the only way to diagnose disc herniation was indirectly with X-rays. As the discs could not be identified, much less the surrounding nerves radiologists relied on noting the spaces between the vertebral bodies; excessively narrow spaces gave doctors a reason to suspect disc herniation.

As contrast medium technology advanced, medical professionals were able to obtain more detailed images of the discs. Contrast medium, a radiopaque material, is injected into the spinal canal before X-ray images are taken. Areas that are compressed by protruding discs appear dark in the images because the fluorescent contrast medium is displaced. This method is called myelogram and has associated risks. It is an invasive procedure and some patients display allergic reactions to the contrast medium. Since there have been some deaths related to myelogram in the past, the procedure is used only when absolutely necessary.

The introduction of MRI technology provides much more detailed imaging of the discs and surrounding structures. In addition to vertebral bodies, MRI images can also clearly show the conditions of the discs, nerves, joints, and ligaments. They reveal the degree of disc rupture and herniation, as well as nerve compressions, and the state of the ligaments surrounding the spines.

MRI imaging of patients that only received non-invasive treatments proved that non-surgical methods not only reduced pain levels, but also improved the physical appearance of the discs. At Jaseng Hospital of Korean Medicine, patients undergo MRI scanning before and after they receive Korean medicine treatments. Most patients' images show that their ruptured discs significantly reduced in size and/or that the ruptured portions disappeared completely. These serial images provide evidence that ruptured and/or protruding discs can be effectively treated without surgery.

Korean Medicine Treatment Has Thousands of Years of Clinical Proof

During the 1980s when the formula of "disc herniation = surgery" dominated the medical community, many people did not readily admit that there could be alternative treatments besides surgery that could reduce the discomfort caused by herniated discs. In particular, many people thought that Korean medicine could not treat these conditions.

Dr. Joon-Shik Shin of Jaseng Hospital of Korean Medicine adamantly refuted this erroneous belief. Having witnessed numerous clinical cases in which disc herniation was healed with only Korean medicine treatment, Dr. Shin wanted to actively promote the effects of his approach.

Conventional medical professionals, however, did not believe that Korean medicine methods could effectively treat disc herniation, saying that there was no scientific evidence. Since thousands of years ago, Koreans have been treating back pain using Korean medicine methods. From our perspective, conventional medicine treatments actually seem comparatively less tested because they have not been used nearly as long.

For many medical problems or diseases, conventional medicine looks to pharmacotherapeutics to find a treatment and then conducts experiments to develop the scientific proof. For example, when a medical agent seems suitable to treat a disease, conventional medicine conducts cell and animal experiments to reveal its effects. If the tests are successful, clinical trials are initiated. However, even after clinical trials, widespread use can reveal previously undetected side effects. As an example, anti-inflammatory drugs, commonly used to treat back pain, were found to increase the risk of cardiovascular diseases and digestive problems. Treatments in conventional medicine include finding solutions to such side effects.

As such, any drug or treatment requires significant amounts of time to prove its safety or effectiveness. Korean medicine has been conducting this validation process for the past several thousand years. For thousands of years, Korean medicine doctors have used various herbal medicines to treat hundreds of thousands of patients, obtaining empirical knowledge about which herbal medicines are effective for various types of diseases.

Traditional treatments demonstrating only a few side effects for thousands of years continue to be used to this day. As such, it is not an exaggeration to assert that there are no safer and more effective treatments than those found in Korean medicine.

Disc herniation is a disease that has plagued humankind since we have started walking upright. Korean medicine treatments for disc herniation have existed for many thousands of years, and in the course of history, they have developed to become more and more effective. It is natural and not unexpected, that Korean medicine provides effective treatments for disc herniation today.

2. Jaseng Treatment does 80% of the Work; Patient Initiative does 20%

"Will the Treatment Completely Cure Me?"

There are two types of patients who visit Jaseng Hospital of Korean Medicine. The first type of patient knows very well that they have disc herniation. In general, they have suffered from disc herniation for a relatively long period of time and often have received a couple of surgery recommendations from other hospitals. They visit Jaseng because they do not wish to undergo surgery.

The second type of patient learned that they have disc herniation after visiting our hospital for a sore back or other minor symptoms. They had not considered that they could have disc herniation, and the narrowed space between their vertebral bones only became apparent after obtaining X-rays. Later, MRI scans of these patients often reveal the advanced degree of disc herniation that had progressed significantly before seeking Korean medicine treatment.

Regardless of whether they are the first or second type, all patients commonly ask if they will be healed completely after receiving treatment. As medical professionals, we wish that we could tell the patients that they will be 100% cured after treatment, however the reality is that we cannot provide the answer that all patients desperately seek.

Disc herniation can be improved when patients receive appropriate and adequate treatment after an accurate diagnosis. Some patients who visit Jaseng express doubt, often asking if they absolutely need MRI scans. From the doctor's perspective, MRI images serve as important evidence that establsihes the extent of disc herniation and which treatment needs to be provided. MRI images can provide an accurate determination, as to whether only pain treatment is required or if long-term preventive care will be required. Furthermore, such images can help differentiate whether the cause of pain is from disc herniation or from other diseases.

For example, if the patient is experiencing severe pain without evidence of disc herniation on the MRI scan, the diagnosis is simply muscular soreness and only pain treatment is required. It is sufficient to stop the pain through Chuna manual therapy or acupuncture, and then restore balance in the patient's back. There is no need to pursue further treatment once the pain subsides

On the other hand, even if the patient has complained only of mild soreness in the back, if the MRI scans reveal disc herniation, then treatments for both the pain and the disc herniation are required. If the discs and nerves have been damaged, or if the surrounding ligaments have been weakened, herbal medicine may be prescribed to supply more nutrition to the discs.

As explained, providing adequate treatment tailored to the specific condition of the patient will lead to the improvement of disc herniation symptoms. However, even optimally designed treatments cannot completely restore damaged discs to their original condition.

Jaseng treatments can restore about 80% of original disc functionality.

The recovery of the remaining 20% of functionality depends on the patients' efforts. Disc herniation is mostly caused by poor lifestyle habits. It is through modifying these habits that patients are responsible for the remaining 20% of their recovery. Even when Jaseng treatments can the pain to subside and restore disc functionality, disc herniation can recur if the patient continues the bad habits that place stress on the spine.

Many people have the misconception that disc herniation is a disease caused suddenly by bursts of strenuous activities. However, disc herniation is the result of continued weakening and degeneration of back structures over time. Although there are patients who develop disc conditions caused by traffic accidents or falling, such cases account for less than one percent of all disc herniations. Since most disc herniations do not occur acutely, time is needed for damaged discs to properly heal. A complete cure is only possible when disc herniation is properly understood and the patient makes continued efforts to manage the condition.

Lack of Pain Does not Mean Complete Recovery

"For the past ten years, I have suffered from intolerable pain for 2 weeks a year. Then the pain would magically disappear for a while. Right now, I don't feel any pain, but I came to the hospital because I want to manage my condition when I don't feel sick."

Said Gyeong-mi Kim (female, age 43) when she first visited Jaseng Hospital of Korean Medicine. She did not want to suffer from pain anymore and asked us to uproot the disc herniation through treatments.

Doctors are often challenged when they are tasked with treating patients who are asymptomatic at the time of presentation. This is because it is difficult for the doctor and the patient to reach a consensus. Patients with severe pain become satisfied with treatment when their pain subsides. It is often difficult for doctors to determine how to treat patients who do not have pain.

Because Jaseng treatments do not involve surgery or injure the muscles, there is nothing harmful about the treatments. However, providing the same treatment all the time can result in different levels of satisfaction for each patient.

Fortunately, Ms. Kim was well aware that treatment would take a long time because she had been through extended periods of pain. Ms. Kim's doctor had extensive discussions with her to reach an agreement about the direction of her treatment.

Since Ms. Kim had been suffering from severe pain for around 2 weeks every year, she was curious if the standards for being "cured" would be absence of pain for over a year and if she could manage her condition at home after that point. Since disc patients often maintain habits that put stress on their back, there always exists the possibility that disc herniation will recur.

Recurrence may not take place, but doctors cannot confidently say that their patients will be "cured," because it is a matter of probability.

To Ms. Kim's question, the doctor answered, "Right now, your discs have only 20 to 30% of their original functionality in absorbing shock and protecting the back. Your disc herniation has been worsening gradually every year, causing you significant pain. Fortunately, the inflammation in the damaged discs that is mainly causing the pain can be treated relatively quickly. That is why your pain did not last for more than 2 weeks at a time. As such, you need treatment that will strengthen your discs and back muscles to prevent the progression of the disc herniation, and it is important for you to change your life habits. Pain is a warning sign that your body sends as the disease worsens."

The doctor told Ms. Kim about the importance of continued treatment and management of the condition. Fortunately, because Ms. Kim had first visited Jaseng after lengthy and repeated bursts of pain, she easily understood the necessity of relatively long-term treatment and management.

Disc herniation is not cured just because the pain caused by the condition subsides. In order to prevent recurrences, the patient needs to continue receiving Chuna manual therapy to correct the physical structure of the back, keep taking herbal medicine to supply nutrition to the discs and the spinal ligaments and muscles, and maintain good lifestyle habits for the discs.

At least 3 months are required for the constitution of the body to change. Because Ms. Kim was not in pain when she visited the hospital, the doctor decided not to prescribe pain treatment, instead focusing on treatments that prevented the progression of disc herniation. Thanks to more than 3 months of persistent treatment, Ms. Kim did not experience back pain for 3 years after treatment. Even though her disc herniation has improved, Mr. Kim still visits Jaseng 2 weeks every year to receive Korean medicine non-invasive treatments and to manage her back condition.

Diseases such as disc herniation that do not heal quickly must be treated by harnessing the self-healing power of the human body through natural physiological processes. Treatments provided by Jaseng Hospital of Korean Medicine aim to stimulate the self-healing power of the human body. When patients foster their bodies' self-healing abilities with the aid of Jaseng treatments and reduce stress on their spines through good life habits, they will be able to fully cure their disc herniation conditions.

3. Shinbaro Herbal Medicine: The Core of Non-Invasive Korean Medicine Treatment

Shinbaro Herbal Medicine, the Scientific Product of Chungpa-jun

"How can herbal medicine remove protruding discs? It doesn't stimulate the discs with needles and it doesn't directly correct the posture. Is it really effective?"

Disc patients who visit Jaseng Hospital of Korean Medicine often have difficulty understanding the effectiveness of herbal medicine. Of course, people who are new to Korean medicine are also doubtful of acupuncture and Chuna manual therapy. However, most people believe that acupuncture and Chuna manual therapy are more effective treatments for disc herniation than herbal medicine. This is because the common perception is that acupuncture reduces pain and Chuna manual therapy corrects the position of distorted bones and muscles, which can help with disc herniation symptoms.

Patients nowadays are well-informed

That is why they do not want treatments offered by doctors if they do not understand them. Doctors must provide sufficient explanations to doubtful patients if they wish to persuade them of the effectiveness of treatment.

"Herbal medicine is a more effective and more direct treatment for disc herniation. Think about acupuncture. Even the needles that penetrate the deepest parts cannot reach the discs. Herbal medicine, on the other hand, is absorbed and then travels through the blood vessels to reach the damaged soft tissues around the discs. If you take herbal medicine persistently, it will be able to effectively treat disc herniation."

Among the non-invasive treatments offered by Jaseng, Shinbaro herbal medicine is a core treatment method that works to help damaged discs recover and strengthens weakened muscles and ligaments, thereby alleviating the conditions associated with disc herniation. Shinbaro herbal medicine was developed from Chungpa-jun, a creation of the late father of Dr. Joon-Shik Shin. Chungpa-jun is an herbal medicine with properties for treating disc conditions that have been scientifically proven.

In 1990, Dr. Joon-Shik Shin was featured on the KBS TV program "Ask Us Anything" and presented a lecture on disc diseases. The public response was explosive. After learning that disc herniation could be treated without surgery and with Korean medicine treatments, people began visiting Jaseng Korean Medicine Clinic (located in Yeoksam-dong from 1990 to 1999; expanded and renamed to Jaseng Hospital of Korean Medicine in July 1999 and relocated to Apgujeong; further expanded and relocated to Nonhyeon in 2017). In addition, word-of-mouth traveled quickly and the hospital attracted even more disc disorder patients. Because of the increased volume of patients, Dr. Shin did not have the time to administer Chuna manual therapy to them all. He often prescribed herbal medicine, leaving Chuna treatment to other doctors.

In addition, there was not enough time to decoct the herbal medicine at the hospital. The patients were instructed to decoct the herbal ingredients in a brew at home, and then drink the decocted medicine for one month before visiting the hospital. Reservation rates soared during those years.

One patient said, "It's just amazing. Even after countless treatments elsewhere, my discs did not get better, but I feel so much better after taking herbal medicine."

Even though most patients received only one session of Chuna manual therapy and took herbal medicine at home for a month, most of them saw improvements in their conditions. Even patients who received diagnoses for severe disc herniation that were told that they would require surgery at conventional medicine hospitals saw tremendous results from herbal medicine.

Some patients, however, complained about having to take herbal medicine, saying that they only wanted to receive Chuna manual therapy as it had been featured on TV. Every time he heard such complaints, Dr. Shin patiently explained that herbal medicine is required to treat the fundamental cause of disc herniation. When patients understood the need for herbal medicine, they began to show better compliance, and these led to more satisfactory results. Over time, these patients became strong supporters of herbal medicine treatment for disc herniation.

Spine medicine circles and the medical community at the time, however, was not happy about Dr. Shin's approach. Even when people who had been diagnosed with severe disc herniation supposedly requiring surgery improved after taking Chungpa-jun, the medical community continued to express its doubts: "How can disc herniation be treated with herbal medicine? It's either placebo effect or a downright lie."

Chungpa-jun, which is the main type of Shinbaro herbal medicine, was developed by the father of Dr. Shin. Chungpa-jun is based on ancient medical texts like Dongeui-Bogam. It contains herbal ingredients that are effective against disc herniation. Al-

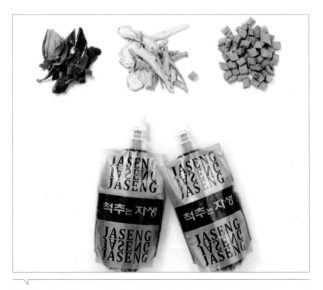

Shinbaro herbal medicine is highly effective against spinal diseases such as disc herniation and spinal stenosis, and its effects have been scientifically proven.

though the effectiveness of the prescription had been known through experience for thousands of years and its effects had been proven empirically in clinical practice, many people still criticized Chungpa-jun for being unscientific and continued to express their disbelief. In response, Dr. Shin decided to scientifically study and prove the safety and effectiveness of Chungpa-jun.

Because Korea was experiencing an economic recession at the time, it was difficult for Dr. Shin to found a research center. Despite difficult conditions, Dr. Shin invested 3.6 billion won to establish Jaseng Research Institute of Biotechnology & Bioscience, which conducted joint studies with the Seoul National University Natural Products Research Institute to analyze the components and mechanisms of Chungpa-jun that were responsible for its effectiveness.

The main ingredients of Chungpa-jun are bangpung, gucheok, duchung, ogapi, and heukdu. The research revealed in addition to these six ingredients, a component in gucheok that had been previously been unknown. That component was named Shinbarometin, which homonymically can mean, "Dr. Shin corrects the spine to an upright position."

Shinbaro herbal medicine is the result of a scientific development project to improve the functionality of Chungpa-jun, a traditional Korean medicine. Since the effects of Shinbaro herbal medicine have been scientifically proven, no one openly doubts the positive effects of herbal medicine on spinal conditions. Shinbaro herbal medicine is effective in combating not only disc herniation, but also other spinal diseases such as spinal stenosis and degenerative disc disorders. As such, it will continue playing a key role in the non-invasive treatments provided by Jaseng.

Scientifically-Proven Effects of Shinbaro Herbal Medicine -Anti-inflammation, nerve regeneration, cartilage protection

After it was promoted to a hospital of Korean medicine in 1999, Jaseng established an independent research center to continue efforts to scientifically prove the effectiveness of Jaseng treatments.

Since 1999, the effects of Shinbaro herbal medicine have been confirmed through various research efforts. The following are some of the key results published in international academic journals.

In 2010, Jaseng worked with Ewha Women's University School of Pharmacy and Seoul National University Natural Products Research Institute to study the anti-inflammatory effects and mechanisms of Shinbaro herbal medicine. To confirm the anti-inflammatory effects of the medicine, the research team divided symptoms into those caused by acute and chronic inflammation since the two types of inflammation involve different cellular responses and enzymes.

To study the responses to acute inflammation, the research team induced inflammation in mice and then injected Shinbaro herbal medicine into one group and provided indomethacin — a commonly prescribed anti-inflammatory drug — for the other group. The experiment found that Shinbaro herbal medicine inhibited enzymes that

Experiment on reduction of inflammation and edema

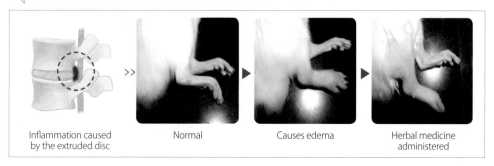

| Inflammation caused by the extruded disc | Normal | Causes edema | Herbal medicine administered |

Mice with inflammation in their feet recovered to normal conditions after they were administered with Shinbaro herbal medicine.

Nerve Cell Process Regeneration Experiment

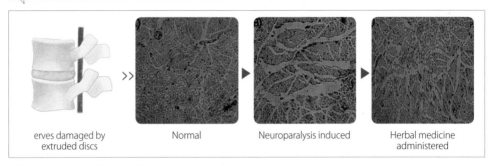

| erves damaged by extruded discs | Normal | Neuroparalysis induced | Herbal medicine administered |

After administering Shinbaro Herbal Medicine in the nerve cells that were induced to have neuroparalysis, the nerve cell processes were regenerated almost to a normal condition.

promote inflammation. In higher doses, it performed as well as indomethacin did.

To study the effects of chronic inflammation, the research team administered Shinbaro herbal medicine for 20 days to mice with induced arthritis, a typical chronic inflammatory disease. The study noted that, the formation of pus and granuloma, commonly associated with chronic inflammation, was inhibited.

Shinbaro herbal medicine was found to be effective against not only acute inflammation, but also chronic inflammation. Extruded discs induce inflammation in the surrounding tissues. Such inflammation also chemically damages nearby nerves, which causes severe pain and functional degradation, ultimately leading to the deterioration of motor functions and senses. Shinbaro herbal medicine has been proven to effectively reduce inflammation caused by disc extrusion.

Shinbaro herbal medicine is also effective in recovering degraded nerve functions. Jaseng conducted joint research with Sungkyunkwan University School of Pharmacy for 10 months, beginning in January of 2009.

In the study, researchers conducted in vivo experiments using mice whose sciatic nerves had been excised, and another set of in vitro experiments using damaged human neuroblasts (SH-SY5Y).

Mice with damaged sciatic nerves had notable difficulty moving one leg. After Shinbaro herbal medicine was administered, the damaged neural functionality began

Cartilage Cell Regeneration Experiment

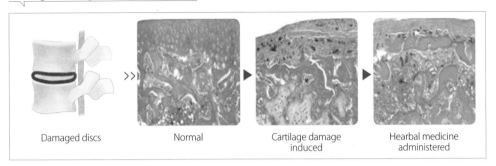

| Damaged discs | Normal | Cartilage damage induced | Hearbal medicine administered |

When mice that were induced to have cartilage damage were administered with Shinbaro herbal medicine, the cartilages were restored almost to a normal condition.

to recover after 2 weeks. After 8 weeks passed, the mice's nerve cells recovered 3 times faster than mice who were not administered Shinbaro herbal medicine. The experiment results also showed that the lengths of the nerves increased as well.

In another experiment, human neuroblasts were oxidatively damaged. The amounts of ROS and LDH that were activated upon cell damage and cell survival rates were measured. In cells treated with Shinbaro herbal medicine, there was a significantly lower concentration of the components that stimulate cell damage, leading to higher cell survival rates.

These studies not only confirm the effect of Shinbaro Herbal Medicine in reducing inflammatory responses caused by disc herniation, but also its ability to actively restore damaged nerves.

To study the ability of Shinbaro herbal medicine to protect cartilage, the Jaseng Hospital of Korean Medicine and Sungkyunkwan University School of Pharmacy research teams induced osteoarthritis in rabbits.

Osteoarthritis damages cartilage and induces the secretion of glycosaminoglycan (GAG). The effects f Shinbaro herbal medicine were compared with those of diclofenac, an analgesic anti-inflammatory drug used to treat bone and joint diseases. Both groups of rabbits experienced inhibition of GAG secretion. Also, in an experiment using the joints of mice, the cartilage density was observed in the subjects following 28 days of oral administration of Shinbaro herbal medicine. Cartilage tissues from the mice that were administered Shinbaro herbal medicine were restored; the experimental group's cartilage tissues were denser than those of mice that did not receive the medicine.

Shinbaro herbal medicine is effective against spinal diseases and safe for long-term administration. In general, herbal medicine is taken for longer periods of time, typically between 6 and 12 months. Taking analgesic medicine for that much time may damage the stomach and increase the liver somatic index. Many international studies have reported that sustained administration of analgesics can cause cardiovascular diseases such as stroke and myocardial infarction.

How about Shinbaro herbal medicine? In general, people are concerned about the liver toxicity of herbal medicine, but such worries are unfounded. Jaseng Hospital of Korean Medicine analyzed 6,894 patients to study the prevalence of liver toxicity problems associated with Shinbaro herbal medicine. The study did not reveal any toxicity issues that could be traced back to the herbal medicine.

Of note, patients with liver toxicity induced by the chronic use of analgesics administered by other hospitals before coming to Jaseng demonstrated lower liver somatic index values after starting Shinbaro herbal medicine.

Of note, 60% of patients who had preexisting liver toxicity issues had their problems subside after taking herbal medicine. Because the study was the largest analysis of patients with liver toxicity subsequently started on Shinbaro herbal medicine, the study was published in an international academic journal.

Why, then, does the false association of liver toxicity with herbal medicine persist in Korea? This may be because of certain interests surrounding the issue. One of the largest studies on liver diseases published in Korea reported that 12 out of 100,000 patients suffer from liver damage caused by drugs (both conventional drugs and herbal medicine). Such statistics are not significantly different from comparable data from other countries. In France, drug-induced liver injury occurs in 13.9 patients per 100,000 patients, and the number is 19.1 patients per 100,000 in Iceland. As such, data relating to drug-induced liver injury should be similar in Korea when compared to that of other countries, but that is not the case: In Korea, 27.5% of drug-induced liver injury is attributed to herbal medicine while 27.3% is linked to conventional medication.

Such distribution is different in Japan, where conventional medicine doctors are allowed to prescribe herbal medicine, thus reducing any conflicts of interest between stakeholders of conventional medicine and herbal medicine. In Japan, 70% of doctors are said to prescribe herbal medicine. According to a report that tracked cases for 10 years in Japan, 60% of all drug-induced liver injury was caused by conventional medicine. In contrast, only 7.1% of drug-induced liver injury was found to have been caused by herbal medicine. Herbal medicines cause problems at only a tenth of the frequency of conventional medicine, which clearly indicates the better safety profile of herbal medicine.

After various studies that scientifically proved the effectiveness and safety of Shinbaro herbal medicine, the spinal medicine community has lessened its skepticism about herbal medicine. Shinbaro herbal medicine is an outstanding treatment that deters inflammation, regenerates bones and nerves, and protects cartilages, ultimately improving the self-healing abilities of the human body. Moreover, long-term administration of herbal medicine does not cause issues associated with liver toxicity. It is clearly a safe and effective non-invasive treatment that can be recommended to many disc herniation patients.

Shinbarometin:
The Core Ingredient of Shinbaro Herbal Medicine

Shinbarometin was discovered in the process of researching Chungpa-jun, a substance made from the extracts of many herbal ingredients. Shinbarometin treats spine, bone, and joint diseases. Animal experiments, as well as cellular and molecular biology experiments identified that Shinbarometin deters the proliferation of cells that cause bone and joint diseases, in addition to its ability to effectively regenerate nerve cells.

After discovering Shinbarometin, Jaseng Hospital of Korean Medicine applied for patents in Korea, Japan, and the U.S (patent acquired in 2003). The U.S. patent for this herbal medicinal agent—with properties that can regenerate bone—was particularly notable, since the U.S. is known for its strict and rigorous patent granting process regarding pharmaceuticals.

Despite positive treatment outcomes, herbal medicines have been ostracized by the conventional medical community because of a lack of scientific proof regarding their mechanisms.

After the effects of Shinbarometin was scientifically proven, Jaseng began developing a new drug containing Shinbarometin in collaboration with GreenCross pharmaceuticals.

After 8 years of research, GreenCross developed Shinbaro Capsule, in January 2011. Clinical trials were held in 8 university hospitals, including Gangnam St. Mary's Hospital and Severance Hospital in Sinchon, with astounding results.

Shinbaro capsule was found to have anti-inflammatory effects comparable to those of Celebrex (component name Celecoxib), the most widely used arthritis drug in the world. In addition, Shinbarometin was found to have little to no adverse effects.

Currently, Shinbaro capsule is available on the market as the No. 4 new natural product-derived drug in Korea (in order of development). The conventional medicine community in Korea, which has historically denied the effectiveness of herbal medicine, currently prescribes prescription drugs based on Shinbarometin, the core component of Shinbaro herbal medicine.

Shinbaro Pharmacopuncture: Acupuncture Delivery of Shinbarometin

The pain relieving effects of acupuncture are well known. The new back pain guidelines published by the American College of Physicians recommend using non-pharmacological treatments before initiating pharmacological treatments.

The publication mentions acupuncture as one such non-pharmacological treatment for use in acute, subacute, and chronic low back pain.

Acupuncture research suggests that stimulating areas experiencing pain induces the brain to secrete opioids, which are narcotic analgesics. In addition, acupuncture can relax tense muscles.

Pharmacopuncture is a combination of acupuncture and herbal medicine, providing a synergistic effect of the two treatments. Components in herbal medicine are injected through acupuncture needles to reduce pain and strengthen the weakened bones, joints, muscles, and ligaments.

In pharmacopuncture, components extracted from herbal medicine ingredients, such as deer antler, ginseng, safflower, and bee sting, are used.

Jaseng Hospital of Korean Medicine developed Shinbaro pharmacopuncture using Shinbarometin. The effects appear more quickly than any other type of pharmacopuncture needles. Patients admitted to Jaseng were administered with either regular pharmacopuncture or Shinbaro pharmacopuncture in a study. The group that received Shinbaro pharmacopuncture treatment recovered much more quickly.

Directly injecting Shinbaro pharmacopuncture in the acupuncture point of the area causing pain enables effective treatment of severe disc herniation patients whose conditions have not improved despite lengthy treatment processes.

Furthermore, pharmacopuncture treatment is useful for patients who cannot tolerate oral medicine for various reasons. There are many cases in which patients who

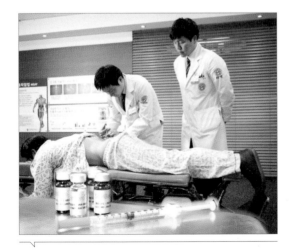

Made with Shinbarometin, Shinbaro pharmacopuncture is faster and more effective than regular pharmacopuncture treatments. Also, it is useful for patients who cannot take herbal medicine.

Jaseng Bee Venom Pharmacopuncture Therapy

Bbee venom therapy uses refined bee venom injected into acupuncture points. The mild heat and immune reaction observed after bee venom acupuncture is similar to the effects of moxibustion. The combination of effects generated by acupuncture and moxibustion alleviates pain or inflammation that may not be effectively treated by regular acupuncture treatment.

The effects of a single session of bee venom therapy can last from 3 to 7 days, making it an economically efficient choice. However, patients must undergo a test to determine whether they are hypersensitive to bee venom. Even after testing negative in allergy exams, patients who receive bee venom therapy may experience soreness, fever, chills, and swelling of the body for 2 to 3 days following treatment.

As explained, despite the high effectiveness of bee venom therapy, it can cause discomfort and mild side effects in hypersensitive patients. For these reasons, patients tend not to prefer this treatment. To solve this problem, Jaseng Hospital of Korean Medicine has removed histamine and other possible side-effect inducing components from bee venom to improve the substance's safety.

An experiment comparing the effects of regular bee venom acupuncture and Jaseng bee venom acupuncture was conducted in 2015. The results showed that while the anti-inflammatory effects were the same, the method used by Jaseng had significantly less skin hypersensitivity reactions. Some patients who received regular bee venom therapy experienced swelling and itchiness, but these symptoms rarely appeared in those who received Jaseng bee venom therapy. The differences in effects were recognized by the Journal of Ethnopharmacology, an international academic journal that published the results noting the safety of Jaseng bee venom therapy.

In clinical practice, bee venom therapy is often combined with Shinbaro pharmacopuncture, rather than alone. Bee venom therapy is applied as needed while conducting Shinbaro pharmacopuncture.

When the two treatment methods are used appropriately, inflammation and pain can be effectively reduced and the immune system can be enhanced, ultimately resulting in a quicker resolution of f disc conditions.

cannot herbal medicine because of their weak digestive systems have experienced improvements in their back disc conditions after receiving Shinbaro pharmacopuncture treatment.

More than anything, Shinbaro pharmacopuncture is attractive in that it can reduce pain without side effects and can effectively treat disc herniation. Bee sting therapy, which is reported to be highly effective in treating spine and bone diseases, also causes hypersensitivity in some patients. Shinbaro pharmacopuncture, however, rarely causes hypersensitivity and patients can receive therapy safely. Shinmarometin utilized in Shinbaro pharmacopuncture not only reduces inflammation, but also regenerates the nerves, cartilages, and bones, providing fundamental treatment of disc herniation.

After the introduction of Shinbaro pharmacopuncture, more successful disc herniation treatment cases were observed at Jaseng. As Shinbaro pharmacopuncture was added to the list of treatments that already included Motion Style Acupuncture Treatment, Chuna manual therapy, and Shinbaro herbal medicine, Jaseng's treatment success rate for disc herniation has climbed to 95%. This indicates that even the most obstinate disc herniation can be effectively treated at Jaseng.

4. Motion Style Acupuncture Treatment (MSAT): Helping Patients Recover Themselves

Can Motion Style Acupuncture Treatment Relieve Paralysis?

Gi-ho Choi (male, age 51), exercised regularly to manage and reduce his symptoms of lumbar stenosis. Despite his extensive efforts, he experienced sharp pains in his back last summer.

For the first 3 days the symptoms were mild, but on the morning of the 4th day, he was not able to get out of bed.

His condition worsened to the point where he could not move his body. He came to the hospital on a stretcher. Mr. Choi complained of severe pain that extended from the tip of his fifth toes to his hips every time he moved his feet. The diagnosis was severe stenosis between the L4 and L5 vertebral elements with a herniated disc in that region that was compressing the nerves.

Chuna manual therapy was administered to correct the structural dysfunctions of the spine. Later, acupuncture needles were applied to five points on Mr. Choi's body. With the needles still in place, Motion Style Acupuncture Treatment was administered by the medical staff, who helped Mr. Choi walk around the halls several times. The goal was to reduce his pain and relax his tightened muscles and ligaments. After 20 minutes, Mr. Choi was able to walk on his own without the help of assistants. In disbelief that he was able to ambulate unassisted, Mr. Choi exclaimed, "Motion Style Acupuncture

Treatment is certainly an effective emergency measure. Because I experienced back pain frequently, I'm used to moving my body in severe pain. This was the first time that I could not move my body at all, as if I was paralyzed. After acupuncture, I can walk without a cane. I can't believe it!"

Patients who receive Motion Style Acupuncture Treatment and their guardians are usually astounded by the patient's quick recovery. It is quite impressive to see an immobile patient stand up and walk after only 20 to 30 minutes of treatment.

How does Motion Style Acupuncture Treatment relax the nearly paralyzed back so quickly?

Patients who arrive at the hospital via ambulance usually cannot move at all. This commonly occurs because the patient's brain has determined that the discs are severely damaged. In response, the brain signals the back muscles to contract and stop moving for protection.

When ligaments or muscles are injured, nearby muscles contract, which applies pressure to the area. The contracting muscles restrict the motion of the joints. When joint motion is restricted, the blood vessels are compressed, affecting blood circulation. When blood flow to an area is reduced, muscles located deep inside the body suffer from lack of oxygen and nutrients, causing extreme pain.

Many people believe that severe pain preventing movement indicates significant damage to the discs, but that is not the case. Even damage that is objectively not serious enough to induce paralysis can lead the brain to send signals for paralytic reactions throughout the body.

For patients whose brains create paralytic reactions in their bodies, Jaseng staff provide physical assistance and support from both sides to help them take measured steps. At first, the patient is fully dependent on the assisting staff, barely moving on their own. Next, the doctor applies acupuncture needles on the points that immediately react to pain. In response, the brain secretes a burst of substances that reduce the level of pain. The patient, initially suffering from intense pain, begins to take small steps on his or her own as the pain subsides.

As the patient walks with assistance, the brain understands that the discs have not

Motion Style Acupuncture Treatment

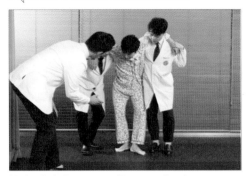

Motion Style Acupuncture Treatment Step 1
The patient is supported by assistants for the treatment.

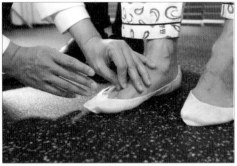

Motion Style Acupuncture Treatment Step 2
Acupuncture needles are applied to 5 points including the back of the neck and the feet.

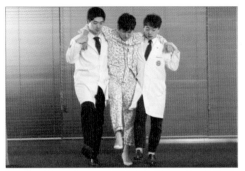

Motion Style Acupuncture Treatment Step 3
Two doctors help the patient ambulate.

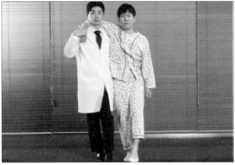

Motion Style Acupuncture Treatment Step 4
As the patient's pain subsides, the level of assistance is decreased.

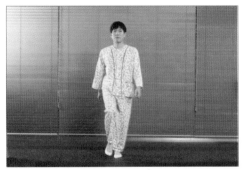

Motion Style Acupuncture Treatment Step 5
The patient is able to walk on his own again.

Walking with the assistance of Motion Style Acupuncture needles in the body reduces the pain and relaxes the tense muscles and ligaments. This is an effective emergency measure that quickly allows nearly-paralyzed patients walk unassisted.

been damaged as severely as assumed. That is when the doctor stimulates the acupuncture needle already in the patient's body, and the brain secretes additional pain-controlling substances. The pain that had decreased from a 100 on a 100 point scale, decreases to a 90, and then to an 80.

Motion Style Acupuncture Treatment, stimulating and relaxing stiffened muscles in the process, pushes the patient to move independently. The treatment also stimulates the muscles that were not used previously, engaging the self-healing power of the body. In practice, there are not many Korean medicine doctors who use Motion Style Acupuncture Treatment on patients experiencing back pain. Patients who experience its effects through therapy however, are motivated which accelerates the treatment process, both for the mind and for the body.

Global Limelight On the Effect of Motion Style Acupuncture Treatment

Motion Style Acupuncture Treatment It is a highly advanced form of acupuncture, manual therapy, and psychotherapy that combines spinal traction, psychological motivation, acupuncture administration, and cognitive therapy.

The effects of Motion Style Acupuncture Treatment often begin within 20 to 30 minutes, which is the time required for patients suffering from extreme pain to get out of their beds and walk around. Unlike acupuncture treatments that require patients to remain motionless in bed, Motion Style Acupuncture Treatment has the patient moving for about 15 minutes with needles inserted in the body. This treatment is most commonly used in emergencies in which movement is restricted, but it is also commonly used to treat symptoms associated with musculoskeletal diseases, such as hip pain, lumbar sprain, and acute sciatic nerve pain.

Along with herbal medicine therapy, Motion Style Acupuncture Treatment is another non-invasive treatment offered by Jaseng. Both are the result of decades-long research conducted by Dr. Joon-Shik Shin. While herbal medicine treats the cause of disc herniation, Motion Style Acupuncture Treatment is a cognitive therapy that quickly induces improvements in patient's symptoms.

As word about the effects of the innovative Motion Style Acupuncture Treatment offered by Jaseng spread, the medical community developed a great interest in its effects. Jaseng Hospital of Korean Medicine worked with the Korea Institute of Oriental Medicine and Pusan National University School of Korean Medicine to study the "Effects and Safety of Motion Style Acupuncture Treatment on Acute Back Pain Patients with Severe Functional Disability."

The study revealed that Motion Style Acupuncture Treatment is effective in providing immediate analgesia and promotes recovery of function in patients with acute back pain and severe functional disorders.

This paper's academic value was recognized when it was published in PAIN (The Journal of the International Association for the Study of Pain), a world-class academic journal.

In the study, 58 back pain patients with severe functional disorders were randomly divided into the experimental group (29 subjects) that received Motion Style Acupuncture Treatment, and the control group (29 subjects) that received muscular injections of non-steroid anti-inflammatory drugs (diclofenac). The reduction in pain and functional disorder improvements of the two groups were evaluated during the study. Before the treatments and 30 minutes after them, the subjects were tested for pain levels in their back and legs (NRS) and spine function disorder index (ODI). Physical tests were also conducted on the lower back. Additionally, the subjects were tested for adverse reactions.

As a result, the group that received Motion Style Acupuncture Treatment experienced less pain in their back and legs 30 minutes after the treatment, and were noted to have lower spine functional disorder index scores. In contrast, the control group reported less pain in the back but not in the legs, and their spine function disorder index was not improved. Also, patients in the experiment group had significant improvements in their physical functions within 30 minutes, enabling them to receive out patient care instead of being admitted to the hospital while the control group experienced little to no improvement that resulted in a hospital stay for 2 to 3 days. In short, the administration of Motion Style Acupuncture Treatment resulted in significant improvements in recovery speed.

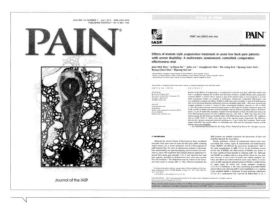

PAIN, where the effects of Motion Style Acupuncture Treatment were published. The cover design symbolized Motion Style Acupuncture Treatment.

The research demonstrated that Motion Style Acupuncture Treatment can immediately reduce the back and leg pain of acute back pain patients and assist in the recovery of spine function disorders at a lower cost. Moreover, the effectiveness of Korean Medicine Treatment was found to be higher than those of anti-inflammatory analgesic injections widely used in conventional medicine.

Many studies report that one of the main mechanisms that converts acute back pain into chronic pain is psychological. Clinical depression and a loss of confidence in recovery turn the condition into a chronic one. This was true regardless of the condition's severity and the length of the time that the patient had been suffering. In this aspect, Motion Style Acupuncture Treatment by producing quick recovery boosts confidence and morale in patients, preventing the disease from becoming chronic.

Motion Style Acupuncture Treatment was introduced through lectures and demonstrations conducted in many foreign medical colleges and university hospitals in the

Dr. Joon-Shik Shin demonstrating Motion Style Acupuncture Treatment to a foreign audience

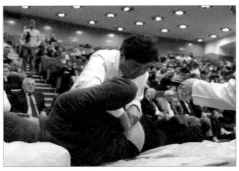

In **2011**, Dr. Joon-Shik Shin was invited by the Russian National Medical School to give a lecture on Jaseng spine treatment methods.

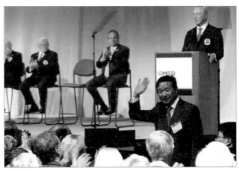

In **2012**, Dr. Joon-Shik Shin was invited to the International Osteopathic Conference in the U.S.

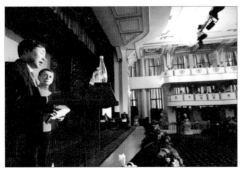

In **2013**, Dr. Joon-Shik Shin was invited by the Kazakhstan National Medical School to give a lecture on Jaseng's non-invasive disc herniation treatment methods.

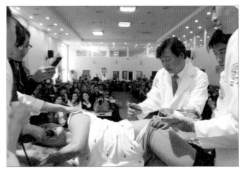

In **2014**, Dr. Joon-Shik Shin was invited by the Mongolia National Hospital No. 3 to give a lecture on Jaseng non-invasive disc herniation treatment methods.

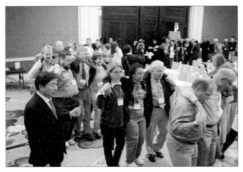

In **2015**, 200 medical professionals from the American Osteopathic Association collectively studied Motion Style Acupuncture Treatment under instruction from Dr. Joon-Shik Shin.

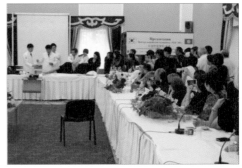

In **2016**, Kyrgyz medical professionals are lsitening to a clinical lecture given by Dr. Joon-Shik Shin at the ceremony celebrating the 70th anniversary of Kyrgyzstan's President Hospital.

U.S., Russia, Kazakhstan, Mongolia, Egypt, and Mexico. Foreign medical professionals continue to show interest in this innovative treatment. In addition to back pain, the treatment is immediately effective in alleviating hip pain, lumbar sprains, and sciatic neuritis. Medical professionals from around the world seek training in Motion Style Acupuncture Treatment. It is also discussed and taught in sessions provided by the American Osteopathic Association (AOA) every year.

5. Chuna Manual Therapy: Restoring Distorted Spine and Muscles

Jaseng, the Origin of Korean Chuna Manual Therapy

"What is Chuna manual therapy? Can it really fix my chronic disc herniation?"

Although Chuna manual therapy has become more common in recent years, people were skeptical when Jaseng Hospital of Korean Medicine first introduced this method to treat disc herniation. Many people were doubtful that distorted bones and joints could be corrected without surgery.

Even though Chuna manual therapy has more than 2,500 years of history, it took a very long for the general public and medical community to recognize that Jaseng's Chuna manual therapy can fix discs without surgery.

Dr. Joon-Shik Shin of Jaseng Hospital of Korean Medicine worked for more than 20 years to develop methods of Chuna manual therapy that can effectively treat disc conditions. Using traditional Chuna manual therapy, he repeated many experiments to find more effective methods, and applied the results to clinical practice to validate the effects.

Although the effects of Chuna manual therapy are now recognized by the conventional medical community, its reaction was not as accepting when the therapy was first introduced. Some medical societies did not recognize the validity of Chuna manual therapy. Nevertheless, Dr. Shin established the Korean Society of Chuna Manual Medicine (currently the Korean Society of

Chuna Manual Medicine for Spine and Nerves), consulting more than 200 academic papers, and conducted various research studies to prove the effects of the method. In the end, he proved that Chuna manual therapy can effectively treat disc conditions without surgery. As the result of many trials and challenges, the Ministry of Health and Welfare is now conducting a pilot project to recognize Chuna manual therapy as an official medical insurance treatment.

Chuna Is a Type of Self-Healing Therapy

The basic principles of Chuna manual therapy are based on the self-healing abilities of the human body. This power is called jaseng-ryuk, or "self-healing power." When the bones and joints in our body shift out of their normal positions, the surrounding blood vessels, ligaments, nerves, membranes, and other soft tissues become swollen.

Chuna manual therapy can be implemented to return the distorted bones and joints to their proper positions. As the bones, muscles, and nearby tissues regain their functions, the pain subsides. This is how Chuna manual therapy works.

The main treatment methods of Chuna manual therapy are "Chu" and "Na." "Chu" is the method of pushing to adjust the bones and muscles, and "Na" is the method of pulling to open up fixed joints and relax soft tissues.

When employing the pushing method, the doctor places the thumbs or palms on the treatment area or acupuncture point to apply pressure in a certain direction to adjust the positions of the bones and joints. This opens up the meridians and facilitates the energy circulation in the body, in addition to dissipating the blood stasis.

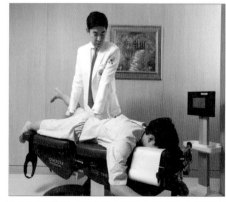

Chuna manual therapy pushes and pulls bones and joints to fix them into their proper places

The pulling method is mainly implemented on the neck, arms, shoulders, and legs. The doctor repeatedly lifts and lowers or pulls on the narrowed joints in the treatment area or at an acupuncture point. The pulling method, which increases the gaps between the bones, is mainly used to treat stenosis, degenerative discs, and other disorders from which elderly people suffer.

As explained, Chuna manual therapy uses pulling and pushing movements to help distorted bones and joints return to their original positions. Because the self-healing power of the body is maximized to treat disc conditions, Chuna manual therapy is safe and effective.

Chuna Can Treat Musculoskeletal System and Internal Diseases

A patient asked, "Doctor, I received Chuna manual therapy for my back pain, and my stomach issues disappeared as well. Before, I experienced indigestion because of stomach problems. I like the improvement, but I still can't believe it. What happened?"

We commonly hear such comments and questions from patients receiving treatment. Chuna manual therapy often not only improves back conditions but also improves digestion and urination, in addition to reducing stuffy feelings in the chest. This is not just a placebo effect.

Although our skeletal structure and internal organs may seem to be entirely separate, they are not. The skeletal structure and internal organs are closely related to each other. In the spine, a thick nerve bundle passes through its center, with the nerves branching out between the bones to connect to the stomach, liver, kidneys, and the heart. When the spinal bones are misaligned and compress the nerves, the body organs inevitably are affected.

The pelvis is also closely related to internal body organs as it contains the urinary bladder, small intestine, and large intestine, as well as the uterus in women. Distorted hip problems can affect these organs.

Chuna manual therapy is commonly conducted on patients with internal diseases.

In Korean medicine, we say that "connection prevents pain while disconnection induces pain." If blood circulation is obstructed, vertebral bones misalign and discs bulge, pressing down on the nerves. When the nerves connected to the stomach are restricted, the stomach suffers, and when those connected to the kidneys are obstructed, the kidneys may experience disease. Chuna manual therapy restores the conditions of the nerves that naturally heal the connected organs.

Patients who have been suffering from disc problems for extended amounts of time will likely suffer from symptoms caused by an imbalance in the internal organs. Chuna manual therapy not only treats disc conditions but also the secondary internal diseases that are the result of the disc conditions.

Patients need to exercise caution after receiving a session of Chuna manual therapy, however. Once distorted, the bones of the spine and surrounding muscles and ligaments often return to their distorted positions even after treatment. This often happens because the muscles and ligaments on one side are already stretched while those on the other side are contracted. Even when the bones are corrected, the muscles and ligaments will often pull and push the bones back into their distorted positions.

As such, it is impossible to correct bones that have become distorted over time with a single session of Chuna manual therapy. Sufficient time must be invested to repeat the treatment procedure multiple times in order to maintain the corrected posture. Also, patients should not rely only on Chuna manual therapy. They themselves must make conscious efforts to fix bad habits and postures that distort the spine.

13 Cases of Herniated Disc Treatment

13 cases of herniated disc treatment and
the accompanying MRI test results are published
with the permission of the individual patients.

Confidence in Treatment Allows Herniated Discs to Pass Like a Cold

Dr. In-Hyuk Ha
(Gangnam Jaseng Hospital of Korean Medicine)

One of the most difficult aspects of treating disc conditions is that patients sometimes do not understand that their conditions can be treated with Korean medicine methods. Significant effort is required on the doctor's part to persuade such patients. If the patient already understands the potential, however, this lengthy process can be easily skipped. Mr. Dong-il Jeong was one such patient who had complete trust in the methods of Korean medicine.

Mr. Jeong (male, in his 60s) was a retired man who often went hiking. He came to me when he experienced pain in his back and legs after hiking about 2 weeks prior. He told me that his discs seemed to have ruptured and requested an MRI scan. Of course, the images revealed that his discs were severely extruded. When I began to explain the causes of disc herniation, how Korean medicine treatments could treat them, and how much improvement he could expect, the patient told me that he was already fully aware of the treatment methods and the effects. He said that he did not need an explanation, and requested inpatient care for his pain.

Normally, patients are extremely curious about their conditions, but Mr. Jeong had surprisingly few questions, which left an impression on me.

Mr. Jeong placed infinite trust in Jaseng's treatments, showing no doubts. All treatments are aided by the placebo effect: Perhaps because of the high level of trust and positive expectations he demonstrated, Mr. Jeong reported that more than 90% of his pain had subsided after 2 weeks of inpatient care. This

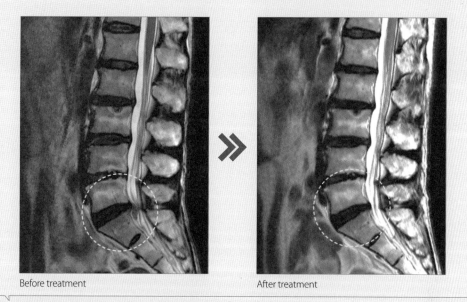

Before treatment

After treatment

Before and after the treatment for the first disc rupture
Inpatient care quickly reduced the pain and the ruptured disc cleanly absorbed back into the body.

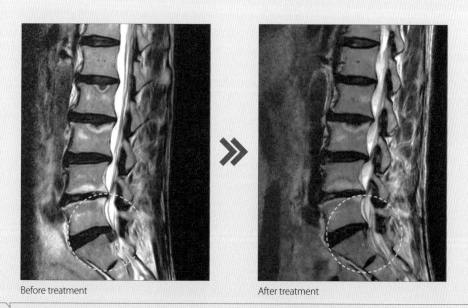

Before treatment

After treatment

Before and after the treatment for the second disc rupture
The disc ruptured again because it was not managed after the first treatment, but it resolved again through Korean medicine treatment.

was a very quick recovery. From my experience, I knew that ruptured discs in patients like him often absorb back into the body. As such, I recommended that an MRI scan be repeated about 2 months later. The MRI images taken 2 months later, revealed that the ruptured discs had resolved.

I remember Mr. Jeong vividly because he did not seem to be very surprised at his fast recovery. I learned later that Mr. Jeong was very familiar with the treatment methods and process of disc absorption because one of his close acquaintances had been treated by me. He later told me that his acquaintance is the reason that he was so confident in his quick recovery.

However, Mr. Jeong did not follow up for additional reinforcement treatments, and his discs ruptured in the same place only 2 years later. He sought inpatient care again, which alleviated his pain within 2 weeks. His discs were reabsorbed in less than 3 months. Some patients recover from a cold within a day or two, but some others suffer for up to a month. Mr. Jeong's discs seemed to rupture easily but also absorb back easily as well, as if he was merely suffering from the common cold. In the end, he was able to overcome his pain and get back on his feet because of his faith in and active cooperation with the Korean Medicine Treatment regimen.

A Patient with Severe Conditions From Russia Returns to Daily Life After Focused, Intensive Treatment

Dr. Ha-neul Kim
(Gangnam Jaseng Hospital of Korean Medicine)

It was the spring of 2017 when Sasha (female, in her 30s) came to visit me from Russia.

In Russia, doctors had recommended that Sasha receive an emergency operation for acute pain in her neck and arms. Diagnostic studies revealed that her discs had severely ruptured and were firmly pressing down on the nerves,. Anxious and fearful of surgery, Sasha chose to receive only nerve injections and pharmacological treatments. The treatments, however, did not alleviate her condition, and because she wanted to avoid surgery, she decided to consult Jaseng after an extensive online search and advice from her acquaintances.

I received her MRI images via e-mail. Her discs were in dire condition. They were not only ruptured, but also pressing down on the nerves very firmly, which made me believe that surgery might be a reasonable option. However, because she was adamantly refusing to undergo surgery, I decided to consult with her through video teleconferencing. During that initial encounter I checked her movements and observed that she showed no severe neurological signs such as loss of arm muscle strength. Since she was only complaining about severe pain, I became certain that I would be able to treat her at the hospital.

After the video teleconference, the patient immediately flew into Korea. Because Sasha lived in the Republic of Khakassia, in the center of Russia where there were no direct flights to Korea, she needed to travel by car for 3 hours to reach the train station, and then travel by train for 5 hours to reach the airport.

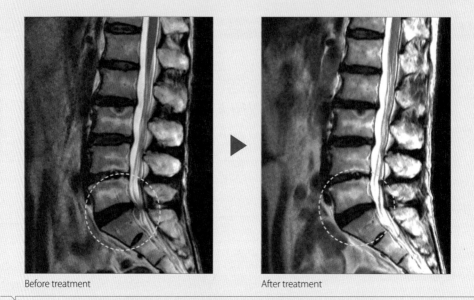

Before treatment   After treatment

Before and after the treatment is given to a Russian patient in her 30's
Although she was recommended to undergo surgery for severe pressure on the nerves, she returned to her everyday routine after 3 weeks of intensive treatment

From there, she took the airplane to complete her 24-hour journey.

I cannot imagine the fear and anxiety she must have felt about going to
a country that she had never been to and where she did not know anyone.
Thinking about the desperation that must have pushed her to overcome such
fears, I firmly resolved to do my best to help her.

The 3 weeks of intensive inpatient treatment began. I conducted thorough
examinations by comparing the patient's conditions and her MRI images, and
then used Shinbaro herbal medicine, Chuna manual therapy, and pharmacopuncture treatment 2 to 3 times a day to reduce the inflammation. Several
days later, the inflammation and arm pain subsided, helping the patient sleep
soundly at night.

When the severe pain had been alleviated, the patient seemed to become
more confident that her body would be able to heal itself. At the end of the 3-week
treatment, more than 80% of her symptoms had resolved. When she returned

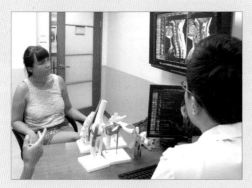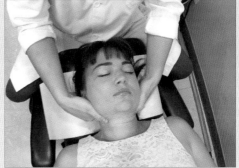

to Russia after her discharge, I prescribed 2 months' worth of Shinbaro herbal medicine.

She returned to the local hospital that had initially diagnosed her and recommended surgery. After reviewing new MRI scan images, the doctors had told her that the results were amazing. Her condition had improved so much that her doctor called her to ask her what treatment she had received to make such a severe disc rupture disappear within 7 months.

Later, Sasha returned to Korea with her husband to treat his back pain and for reinforcement treatments for herself. Reflecting on this patient's clinical course through our non-invasive Korean medicine treatment, as a doctor, I felt indescribably proud.

An Early Pregnant Mother Recovers From Herniated Disc and Successfully Gives Birth, Thanks to Korean Medicine Treatment

Dr. Hae-chan Jeong
(Haeundae Jaseng Hospital of Korean Medicine)

"Doctor, you've got a phone consultation request." A nurse sent me a message via our intranet messenger program.

"Jeong Yeon-hee (age 33). 12 weeks pregnant. Experiencing severe back and leg pain. Took MRI scans in a nearby hospital. Diagnosed with severe disc rupture. No treatment found possible during pregnancy. Requested a phone consultation." The information that caught my eye was that she was 12 weeks pregnant. I thought, "What can I do for this patient?" With a bit of apprehension and a bit of fear, I pressed the phone number.

On the other side of the line, I could hear the desperation of the patient. "Doctor, my pain is so severe that I can't do anything right now. The hospital that tested me said that they can't even use mild painkillers because it's so early in my pregnancy and that they can't use any electric physical therapy. I said that I hesitant about surgery. Do you think I can be treated without surgery?"

I could imagine how great her pain must have been. Most pregnant patients endure their pain and do not receive treatment because they are fearful that medical intervention might be harmful to the child. The pain only worsens, and it becomes more difficult for the patient to endure.

Hoping to help even just in the slightest, I suggested that she visit my office. That same weekend, Ms. Jeong visited my office at Jaseng with her husband and first son. Looking at the medical records she brought, I saw that the disc between the L5 and the S1 vertebra had been severely ruptured. Because of the extreme back pain and tingling in the left leg, it was difficult for her to continue with her daily routine or even walk. Fortunately, because she did not suffer from neurological paralysis, we were able to provide non-invasive treatments using Korean medicine methods suitable for pregnant mothers. We decided to turn to inpatient care. As expected, the patient was concerned that the treatment might adversely affect the fetus. The pain from the ruptured disc, morning sickness, anxiety, and having to leave her first child behind worsened the situation, making the patient suffer psychologically. Because my wife was 4 months pregnant at that time, I sympathized with the patient more than anyone else.

I vowed to myself to do my best to this patient, who had made the difficult decision to seek treatment. I regularly talked to Ms. Jeong and told her about my wife, who took herbal medicine and received pharmacopuncture treatments during her first pregnancy. In fact, my wife, who was going through her second pregnancy at the time, took herbal medicine and received pharmacopuncture whenever she experienced back pain.

The patient's symptoms were alleviated through treatment and the pain became much milder. Although she was unable to walk much at the beginning, she was eventually able to walk for about an hour at a time. After 36 days of inpatient care, the patient returned home. Although her pain had subsided, it seemed difficult for her to let go of the anxiety about having received treatment during pregnancy.

Eight months later, I received very happy news that the patient had given birth to a healthy child.

Today, Ms. Jeong is happily raising her two sons and runs an online store selling children's clothes. She happily complains that her wrists, shoulders, and other joints hurt every time she lifts her second son, who is now over 13 kilograms. I always tell her to remember the difficult treatments she endured, to maintain good postures, and continue exercising.

MRI images of Ms. Jeong completed several days ago to assess her current

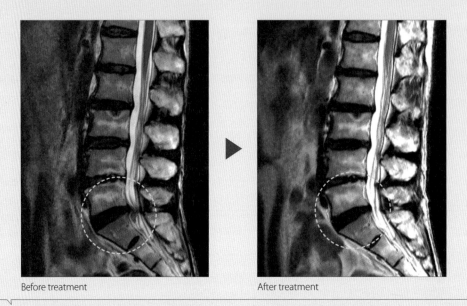

Before treatment

After treatment

Before and after the treatment of a patient in her 30s who visited because her disc ruptured during pregnancy
Inpatient care not only alleviated the symptoms but also led to the healthy birth of her child.

condition show that the ruptured disc which caused her so much physical and psychological pain had absorbed. I am thankful to the mother who trusted my treatment and the baby who trusted his mother to bring him safely into the world.

Constantly Rupturing Discs Absorbed With the Willpower of the Patient

Dr. Jong-hun Park
(Ansan Jaseng Hospital of Korean Medicine)

Sometimes, I lose confidence in the treatment offered to a patient. That was the case with Mr. Ho-jin Jeong (male, age 38).

In November 2014, Mr. Jeong came to my office and talked about the pain in his back and the tingling sensations in his legs that had persisted for the past 3 months. Because his older brother had been suffering for a long time from disc herniation and additional symptoms brought on as a result of back surgery, Mr. Jeong was quite knowledgeable about ruptured discs. He was very aware that his sedentary lifestyle was a primary reason for this condition, and quickly grasped the severity of his symptoms.

MRI scans revealed that the disc between the L4 and L5 lumbar had turned dark, in addition to degenerative changes around the disc.

The disc was protruding I explained to the patient the typical prognosis for the condition and the treatment plan, and initiated outpatient treatments, with the patient visiting the office once or twice every week.

Contrary to my expectations, however, his symptoms did not subside easily after 4 weeks. After the patient and I reached a consensus that this delay was caused because he could not easily correct his lifestyle, I planned an intensive inpatient plan for him. We began inpatient care in December of 2014that included daily procedures as well as doses of Shinbaro herbal medicine.

Despite this intensive inpatient approach, the symptoms did not improve. In fact, his pain levels suddenly increased and the muscle strength in his lower limbs decreased a week into the treatment program. We obtained MRI scans immediately to assess potential causes for the loss of muscle strength. The results were surprising. There was a massive leak of nucleus pulposus around the disc that had only protruded a month earlier. According to the cross-sectional image, the mass covered more than 90% of the spinal canal. Because the symptoms had worsened and the patient's strength had decreased, we needed to be aware of possible cauda equina syndrome. It was difficult to proceed with only Korean medicine treatments. At that point, I recommended surgery to the patient. He adamantly refused. He was resolved to continue on the path of non-invasive treatment. The major reason was that his older brother had continued to experience pain even after he received back surgery. This placed me in a difficult dilemma. Cauda equina syndrome, which can occur following the loss of muscle strength, is an indication that surgery is absolutely required. I tried to persuade the patient many times, but he was adamant that he would postpone the surgery unless the cauda equina symptoms worsened. After a lengthy consultation, we decided to check his muscle strength every day and frequently monitor his urination and defecation functions, as well as monitor for other signs associated with cauda equina syndrome, while continuing his inpatient care routine.

Thankfully, the muscle strength did not progress, and cauda equina syndrome did not develop. To the contrary, the patient reported slightly less pain, indicating a surprisingly quick rate of recovery. Although not much muscle strength returned, the pain quickly subsided over the next 3 weeks of inpatient care. One month into the inpatient program, the patient was discharged as he was well enough to receive outpatient treatments.

I provided more intensive Chuna manual therapy to correct his physical balance and corrected his pathological spine movements. Muscle strength was restored through Shinbaro herbal medicine and pharmacopuncture. After these treatments, the patient's pain subsided enough to enable him to commute to work. We decided to reevaluate the situation 4 months after the initial treat-

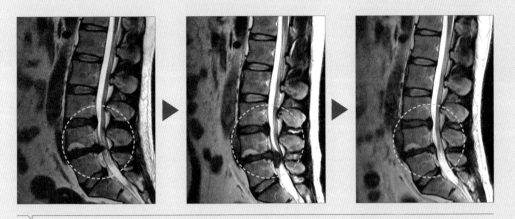

Process of treatment for disc herniation accompanied by back pain and leg tingling
Although the protruded disc ruptured during inpatient care, we continued Korean medicine treatments at the insistence of the patient. The patient has recovered safely and returned to his daily routine.

ment. In April 2015, as expected, the ruptured disc had been significantly absorbed, and more than half of the nucleus pulposus that filled the spinal cavity was gone. We continued additional treatments, and the patient successfully returned to his daily routines.

It is not good practice for a doctor to quickly determine a prognosis or definitively predict the future for a patient. From a medical professional's perspective, I would recommend surgery to a patient whose condition suddenly worsened during inpatient care. However, if the patient is insistent on continuing the current course of treatment and the symptoms are not as clear as they appear in the textbooks, I would definitely draw on this experience to carefully reconsider and consult the patient with an open mind.

Two Surgeries and Three Relapses:
The Malevolent Cycle that was Ended at Jaseng

Dr. Dong-jae Shin
(Bucheon Jaseng Hospital of Korean Medicine)

One summer day in 2014, a female patient walked in with a limp, her face showing obvious pain. The first thing Ms. Ji-eun Choi told me once she sat down was, "Doctor, please fix me. I can't have surgery anymore."

Ms. Choi (female, age 37) was diagnosed with disc extrusion between the L5 and S1 vertebra in the winter of 2013, when she had visited a hospital for pain in her right leg. She had undergone neuroplasty. The pain, however, had not subsided. This led to another surgery. The same disc ruptured again, and the doctor's response was that an artificial disc and pins needed to be implanted into her spine. Determined that she did not want any more surgery, on the advice of acquaintances, she decided to visit Jaseng.

Due to severe pain, she could not sit or stand for even short periods of time, and she could only limp to the bathroom, unable to walk longer. Her pain lessened when she lied down, but it worsened at night, preventing her from sleeping soundly.

Due to the pain, she was noted to have severe scoliosis with a bend to the left side. MRI images indicated that the disc between L5 and S1 was extruded to the right, causing severe pressure on the nerves. The two surgeries had removed the lamina, a part of the spinal structure. The muscles and ligaments surrounding the spine were also damaged and adhesive. Her excessive body weight due to obesity was placing a heavy burden on her back. Further worsening the situation was the despair caused by the third relapse of the condi-

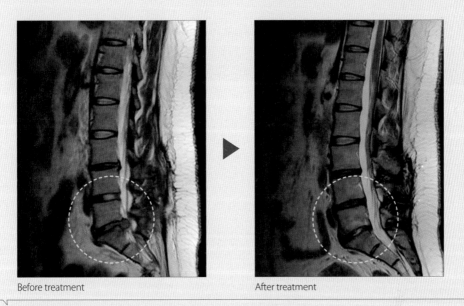

Before treatment   After treatment

Before and after Korean Medicine Treatment for a ruptured disc that did not heal even with two surgeries
After intensive care, the disc recovered to a level that enabled the patient to continue with her daily routine.
The patient is maintaining the treated condition.

tion, as well as the anxiety that she might become permanently disabled. She was also feeling guilt and stress for not having been able to care for her young children for over six months

The fact that there had been 2 surgeries and 3 relapses, the findings on MRI images, the patient's condition, and many other factors indicated that the prognosis was not good. Fortunately, the patient's muscle strength was intact. With the patient's resolve to not have another surgery and with my belief that she might get better with treatment, we decided to admit her.

The pain began subsiding within 3 days of inpatient care. She was able to sleep better at night, and the scoliosis slowly disappeared, which allowed the patient to walk with less of a limp. The patient was gradually able to sit for longer periods, from 3 minutes, to 10 minutes. She was generally very happy with the subsiding pain and her recovering physical functions. I was also happy with the positive treatment results. During about 40 days of inpatient care, her body recovered gradually, the pain was reduced significantly, and the patient was able to carry out some everyday tasks. We decided to treat the remaining symptoms through outpatient care. I was concerned that her symptoms might worsen after she was discharged, but there have been no significant issues since then. After she recovered to the level where she felt no discomfort in her daily routine, we obtained another set of MRI images to check her disc condition. The patient, upon seeing that the disc that was pressing down on the nerves had been absorbed back, bowed down deeply to show her appreciation and cried. Looking at her, I felt proud as well.

Ms. Choi is currently leading a healthy life, caring for her young children. After she was discharged, she needed to be treated again after a traffic accident, but the MRI images indicated that the disc was maintaining a healthy state.

Being able to restore happiness in this patient, I felt great satisfaction in my career as a Korean medicine doctor. Through her case, I am always reminded that I want to help more patients regain their health and happiness.

Herniated Disc During Pregnancy Cured Through Korean Medicine, Allowing Smooth Childcare

Dr. Min-su Kim
(Ansan Jaseng Hospital of Korean Medicine)

When women with back pain become pregnant, the increasing body weight puts more stress on the spine, causing even more severe back pain. Pregnant patients, however, tend to avoid treatment for the sake of the fetus and simply endure the pain. The real problem begins after childbirth. As patients with already weakened backs care for the baby and engage in physically demanding activities, pain will often reach intolerable levels.

Starting from the sixth month of her pregnancy, Ms. Ji-hye Song (age 32) felt pain extending from her back to her right leg, but she endured it until childbirth. As she took care of her newborn baby, the symptoms worsened and she visited a neurosurgeon specializing in spinal treatment. An MRI scan was taken in April of 2017 showed that the disc between the 4th and 5th lumbar vertebra was ruptured; she received a neuroblocking injection. The symptoms seemed to improve after the injection, but the effects were temporary and the pain worsened. She visited another spine hospital. The MRI scan obtained there showed that the nucleus pulposus in the disc was ruptured even more than it had been previously. The doctor advised her that she needed surgery. Because she did not want an operation, she visited many other hospitals searching for other options, but all five doctors she visited recommended surgery

Adamantly opposed to the idea of surgery, the patient continued to seek options until she arrived at Ansan Jaseng Hospital of Korean Medicine. During the first consultation, the patient seemed to be experiencing extreme stress from the constant pain, her childcare duties, and the repeated recommendations for surgery made by the other doctors. Despite the adverse situation, the patient had a strong resolve for non-invasive treatment and displayed a positive attitude about her circumstances. As such, I thought that plenty of rest and treatment would easily lead her to a full recovery.

Ms. Song made the difficult decision of leaving the baby with its father and grandmother to begin an intensive inpatient regimen. Because of her severe pain and fluctuating symptoms, her body did not quickly respond to the treatments. During the second week of inpatient care, the pain near the legs subsided, but the tingling sensation persisted. The pain near the buttocks was especially severe, preventing her from standing for even a few minutes. Fortunately, she had notable willpower and a positive outlook, which allowed her to endure pain as she practiced walking. Although she was apprehensive of

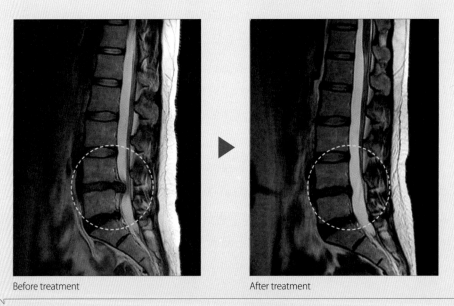

Before treatment   After treatment

Before and after treatment was administered to a patient whose disc rupture that had occurred during pregnancy worsened during childcare
The rupture in the disc between L4 and L5 lumbar vertebra was pressing on the nerves, causing severe pain in the back and right leg. Intensive treatment led the nucleus pulposus to absorb eliminating the pain and pressure on the nerves.

acupuncture needles, she received the recommended treatment without complaint.

Unfortunately, as we began to note improvement in her condition, her mother, who was taking care of the baby, developed pain in her wrists and back that required treatment. The patient had to be discharged to take care of her baby until her mother's condition improved. Fortunately, her symptoms did not worsen during her time back home. When she was readmitted, the treatment progressed much faster. The patient was able to walk for longer periods of time while experiencing less pain.

When MRI images were repeated four months later, she had recovered almost completely. Ms. Song is now able to carry out everyday tasks, travel, and take care of her child without any problems.

I would like to thank the patient who engaged the difficult treatment process with a positive attitude, her mother and husband who sacrificed much during her treatments, and her child who endured time without her mother.

Walking for 2 Hours After a Successful Treatment

Dr. Ji-hun Ahn
(Jamsil Jaseng Hospital of Korean Medicine)

One cloudy day in mid-February, as I was coming down to my office on the 4th floor after lunch. I saw a patient's leg sticking out from behind the wall in the waiting room.

I thought to myself, "Who's lying down like that on the waiting room bench? The patient must be in severe pain."

The patient's guardian was nervously watching the patient, who was lying down with his arm covering his face, groaning in pain.

I thought, "I don't know which doctor will see him, but it won't be easy."

As I walked into my office, a nurse popped in and said, "Doctor, we have a patient with severe pain. I think you'll need to go out to the waiting room to see him."

The patient lying down on the bench had been allocated to my office.

He was not able to get up on his own. When he was helped up, he needed to lie down again almost immediately due to extreme leg pain. Of course, he was not able to carry out everyday tasks. He had to eat lying down, which interfered with his digestion. He was a tall man, well over 185 centimeters. Because he had not been able to walk for a long time due to the pain from disc herniation, he had notable loss of muscle mass, just skin covering the bones like a mummy.

The patient introduced himself as Jae-jin Lee (male, age 40). He had disc procedures twice in October of 2016 for his condition. The procedures were administered in an orthopedic surgeon's office and had done nothing to reduce his pain. When he first spoke to me, Mr. Lee said: "Doctor, I don't care if it takes a lot of time. Please don't let me have surgery."

I could sense the patient's desperation. The MRI images indicated that the disc between the L5 and S1 vertebra was ruptured and was compressing the nerves, preventing the patient from standing for even a full minute. After talking with the patient and his guardian, I decided to admit him to the hospital and immediately begin an intensive treatment program that same day. Beginning with Chuna manual therapy in the morning, the patient also received Shinbaro herbal medicine, nerve root recovery therapy, bee venom therapy, acupuncture treatment, cupping treatment, and physical therapy involving manual treatments. One day, during a nerve root recovery therapy session, the patient asked,

"Doctor, the pharmacopuncture needle seems like it's going toward the area where it tingles and hurts. Is that the right way to do it?"

The patient had been responding well to the nerve root recovery therapy, which involves injecting large doses of Shinbaro pharmacopuncture medicine deep into the damaged nerves with acupuncture needles. After 2 weeks, the patient, who previously was only able to stand for one minute, could remain standing for about eight minutes. He was also able to take small steps with a walker. The pain was reduced by 50% after 1 month of inpatient care. On approximately the 40th day, he was able to walk along the path of the nearby Seokchon Lake for about 30 minutes without assistance. At that point, we discharged him and began outpatient care.

Mr. Lee runs a pig farm in Gyeonggi Province. He has to walk around his farm to maintain the facilities, and he also drives to the market every day.

After suffering from disc herniation for more than six months, he had not been able to manage his farm, much to his distress and anxiety. The patient, however, always walked into my office with a smile and received treatment with a positive attitude.

When patients walk into my office, I always ask about their condition "Mr. Lee, how do you feel today?"

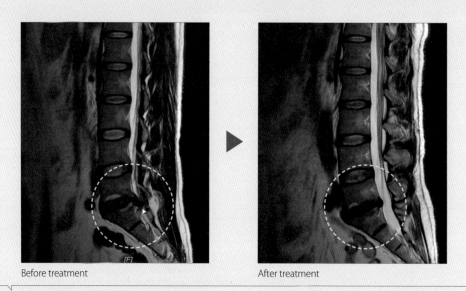

Before treatment · After treatment

Before and after the treatment provided to a patient who could not even stand up
The disc between the L5 and S1 vertebra ruptured and penetrated the posterior longitudinal ligament.
The patient fully recovered after inpatient and outpatient care.

He would always answer, "I feel good. I think I'm getting better."

Mr. Lee always believed that he was getting better, and his hopes became a reality. Whenever I think of Mr. Lee, I am reminded of his thin legs that I saw during his first Chuna manual therapy session. Muscle mass has returned to his buttocks and legs, and he says that people tell him he looks much better after receiving treatment. Stories like this make me feel excited to be a part of the Jaseng medical staff.

After 3 to 4 months of outpatient care, we repeated the MRI scan.

The images showed that the disc had significantly reduced in size. Elated, we congratulated each other. The patient can now walk 2 hours without any problems and leads a normal life.

Every time I see Mr. Lee, it reinforces the idea that a positive mindset and belief in the power of non-invasive treatments to heal ruptured discs works. I walk into my office every day, hoping that I will be able to successfully treat patients suffering from disc herniation without surgery.

Herniated Disc From Hard Work in the Restaurant, Healed Through the Power of Positivity

Dr. Kim Sang-Don
(Haeundae Jaseng Hospital of Korean Medicine)

A thin middle-aged woman with a pale face talked about the severe pain she was experiencing as soon as she walked into my office. It did appear that she was in extreme pain. She touched her calves constantly during the consultation.

Ms. Gyeong-suk Kim (female, age 50) underwent back surgery 2 years ago when her disc ruptured. She visited Jaseng because the pain returned 18 months after the surgery. The pain now was even worse than before. She was taking painkillers and had received several nerve injections, but they had offer minimal relief. She told me that after the pain returned after the surgery 2 years ago, she became afraid of the repeated cycle of surgery and relapse.

Ms. Kim believed that her disc ruptured again because she continued to work at her restaurant—which required her to bend her back frequently I recommended inpatient care because her pain was so severe. I did note that the patient showed a strong resolve to improve her condition.

I have seen countless back disc patients, but cases as severe as Ms. Kim's are rare. For the first 3 weeks after she was admitted, she could not sleep. Despite her relentless pain, Ms. Kim tried to smile and maintain a positive attitude towards her treatment. Every morning, Ms. Kim asked me: "Doctor, I'll get better, won't I? I believe in you and no one else."

I was worried that the treatment might take a long time, but I always answered confidently: "Of course! I've seen worse patients get better. You're not

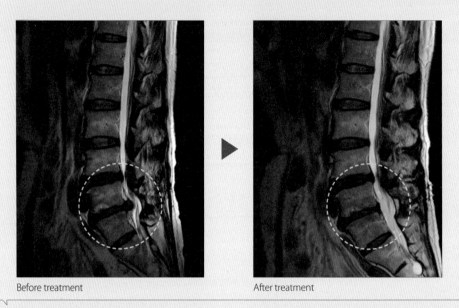

Before treatment　　　　　　　　　　　　After treatment

Before and after the intensive inpatient treatment for a patient whose disc ruptured after surgery
The re-herniated disc reabsorbed cleanly, and the patient recovered to the point in which she could lead a normal daily life.

paralyzed and there are no issues with your bowel movements. You'll definitely get better."

Every morning, the patient and I exchanged the same words.

For the first few weeks, the pain only subsided to a manageable level, and no significant improvement took place. During the 5th week, however, the pain started to ease dramatically. The patient's strong resolve to get better and her positive attitude seemed to have helped.

Patients are always anxious. The same must have been true for Ms. Kim. Thoughts such as "Will the pain last forever?" and "Will I need another operation?" recurred several times a day. Fear and anxiety bind patients in the pitfall of agony. The role of the medical staff is important in this regard. In the process of encouraging patients and caring for them with a tender heart, patients may learn to be less anxious and develop a belief that their condition will improve.

Our brain does not believe the facts. Rather, it believes what it thinks are the facts. Holding on to the conviction that she would get better, Ms. Kim showed slow but sure signs of improvement. She was discharged after six weeks of inpatient care. For the next 3 months, she returned to the hospital weekly for outpatient care.

As she regained her health, she resumed her work at her restaurant as well. MRI images one year later showed that the damaged disc had cleanly reab-sorbed. I was thankful that the patient had managed her condition well after the treatment.

I remember Ms. Kim fondly because she had stronger faith in her complete recovery than I did. Even to this day, she often calls me to say hello, and I some-times visit her restaurant to enjoy a delicious meal.

Patients with disc diseases recoveraided by unwavering trust in their own bodies and a positive attitude.

Experiencing Car Accident During Treatment Helped the Disc Absorb

Dr. Jae-hun Lee
(Daegu Jaseng Hospital of Korean Medicine)

In May of 2016, Ms. Su-jin Jang (female, 30s) came to my office with back pain and tingling in her leg that had appeared several days prior to the visit. The patient was unable to walk even with a support belt around her waist. The diagnosis was a ruptured disc between the L4 and L5 vertebra, causing compression on the nerves. Fortunately, there were no indications of muscle strength deterioration or cauda equina syndrome, which allowed for Korean medicine treatments to be started.

The symptoms rapidly improved. She was able to walk without a support belt within a week, and during the second week, she was able to run errands outside the hospital. I was very happy that the patient was recovering so quickly.

Her relief did not last long. While Ms. Jang was running some errands for her job, she was involved in a car accident.

Minor traffic accidents usually only cause simple stiffness in the muscles. However, because disc patients have weakened muscles and ligaments surrounding the spine, even minor accidents can cause significant problems. As expected, Ms. Jang complained of worse back pains after the accident. I was concerned that the disc being treated might get worse. But I was certain of her recovery because Shinbaro herbal medicine does not simply alleviate the inflammation in the disc, it also strengthens the surrounding muscles and ligaments and regenerates cartilage. I explained to the patient that the regenera-

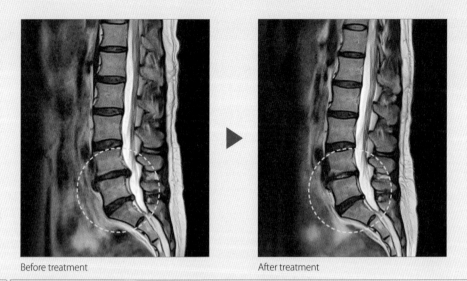

Before treatment   After treatment

Before and after the treatment for a patient who was in a car accident during treatment
During her treatment for a ruptured disc between the L4 and L5 vertebra, the patient was involved in a car accident. The patient recovered without much problem, however.

tive and strengthening properties of Shinbaro herbal medicine would help her recover.

Ms. Jang continued to take Shinbaro herbal medicine during the remainder of her inpatient treatment. As a result, her back pain and the tingling in her leg improved significantly after only 3 weeks (a shorter time frame than anticipated), despite the traffic accident she had suffered. The discs that had been strengthened through the Korean Medicine Treatment must have helped protect her during the accident.

For 3 months after discharge, I directed the patient to continue taking Shinbaro herbal medicine and visit the hospital every 2 weeks.

Exactly 1 year after she was admitted, a repeat MRI scan showed that the ruptured disc had completely reabsorbed.

Korean Medicine Treatment:
The Best Choice of My Life

Dr. Hyeong-cheol Lee
(Gangnam Jaseng Hospital of Korean Medicine)

"All office workers are said to experience back pain at some point due to overwork, office dinners, and bad posture. I was no exception. But because I exercised and stretched regularly to take care of my body, I did not think much of minor back pains. I thought that I didn't need a diagnosis because my pains subsided after a long night's sleep with a hot compress. One day at work, however, I started to experience a numbness and a tingling pain in my right leg. It did not feel like a part of my body and I felt as though I might burst. I had never experienced a pain so severe in my life. Emergency treatments that I was accustomed to performing were of no use, and the pain grew as time passed, preventing me from working or even walking. That's when I dragged myself into a taxi to visit Jaseng Hospital of Korean Medicine."

– Excerpt from Mr. Jun-wu Kim's diary

Mr. Jun-wu Kim (male, age 35) limped into my office, sat down with a stiff look, and asked me to do something about the extreme pain in his leg so that he could return to his office. However, I persuaded him to undergo a thorough examination including an MRI scan.

As I had expected, the disc between the L4 and L5 vertebra was ruptured and impinging on the right side. The images showed some of the most severe situations I had seen. At this stage, most conventional medicine hospitals would recommend surgery. Even at our hospital, we would recommend surgery if no improvements or neurological changes were eventually observed. But because I had seen many cases in which patients who were recommended to have surgery recovered with non-invasive treatments, I told Mr. Kim that 2 to 3 weeks of intensive inpatient care would be the best course of action to alleviate the most severe symptoms.

Mr. Kim responded that his company never allowed sick time and that people who took time off had had to leave the company. He strongly refused my recommendation for inpatient treatment. That began the long process of persuasion. Ultimately, Mr. Kim said that he wanted to avoid surgery if non-invasive treatment was possible, and agreed to begin the inpatient treatment.

That evening, his parents visited my office. I showed them the MRI images and explained the symptoms and the treatment process. The parents were very concerned about their son's condition. The mother was especially distraught and broke into tears.

She said, "I know it is difficult, but if my child needs surgery, please tell us frankly."

I answered, "The symptoms and test results indicate that the condition is serious. We need to see how the situation progresses, it is important that he be admitted for about 2 to 3 weeks. I will do my best to treat him." After my detailed explanation, the parents agreed and returned home.

We immediately began an intensive care regimen involving nerve root recovery therapy and Shinbaro herbal medicine. Day by day, the extreme pain in the leg subsided. With every visit, Mr. Kim asked, "Do the acupuncture needles and herbal medicine have painkilling substances?" His trust in the treatment helped him recover. As promised at the beginning, we discharged the patient once the most severe symptoms were alleviated on the tenth day. Although he could not return to work immediately, Mr. Kim continued receiving outpatient treatments while resting at home. In the beginning, he visited the hospital 2 to 3 times a week, and eventually just once a week. At that point, he returned to

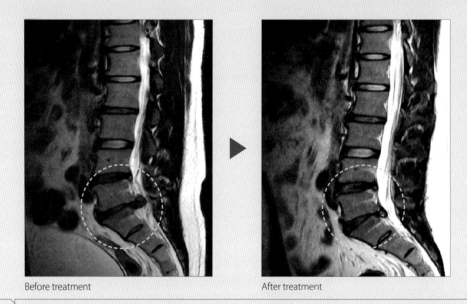

Before treatment　　　　　　　　　　　　　　After treatment

Before and after the treatment for a patient whose disc ruptured due to overwork
The situation was serious enough to warrant surgery. After inpatient treatment, the patient recovered enough to return to work.

work as well.

About 3 months later, his symptoms were almost completely gone. Six months after the first consultation, we performed another series of MRI scans.

The results were extremely satisfactory. Not only were the symptoms alleviated, but the images also indicated that the ruptured disc had significantly re-absorbed

Mr. Kim said that seeking Jaseng's non-invasive treatment was the best choice of his life. He no longer experiences pain. He told me that he will never forget the images of his ruptured and isolated disc. I am extremely proud of this case because it proves that Jaseng's non-invasive spine treatments can not only alleviate the symptoms, but also promotes healing.

Effective Treatment Generates Patient Confidence

Dr. Un-seok Jeong
(Ulsan Jaseng Hospital of Korean Medicine)

I have always thought that doctors should not have preconceived notions or biases concerning their patients. I believed that we should alwyas consider the patients' symptoms and objective diagnoses before conducting appropriate treatments. After encountering various types of patients, however, I started to realize that I was subconsciously building biases. I had been prejudiced to believe that highly educated, white-collar workers tended to trust conventional medicine less and to view Korean medicine with skepticism. The patient that I will discuss fell, in my mind, into this category.

Mr. Ho-yeong Gang (male, age 40) was a naval architect. Because he worked long hours in front of a computer, exceptional stress was placed on his back. Also, the recession in the shipbuilding industry had driven his company to compete with low prices and faster turn-around periods. As a result, Mr. Gang was forced to sit in front of a computer for more than 10 hours a day. Back pain was a natural result.

During his first visit, he complained of severe back pain and numbness in the front part of his left thigh. He was also noted to have a reduced ability to move due to reduced muscle strength.

MRI images indicated that all discs were degenerating, and the one between the L2 and L3 vertebra was severely ruptured, severely compressing the nerves. I could imagine the pain even without the patient telling me about it. Mr. Gang also expected his condition to be bad, but he did not seem to expect it to be so

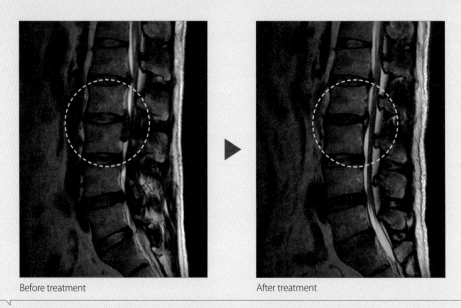

Before treatment   After treatment

Before and after the treatment for a patient who did not trust Korean Eastern medicine
His discs were degenerating and the disc between the L2 and L3 spines was ruptured and pressing down hard on the nerves. After the Korean Eastern treatment, the ruptured disc was cleanly reabsorbed.

severe. Although I explained a detailed treatment plan for him, he was not eas-ily persuaded about the Korean medicine treatments because he believed that surgery was necessary. I emphasized that he was still relatively young, and sug-gested that the 3 months required for treatment was not much time compared to the life ahead of him. I was so adamant because I was confident that I could treat him successfully.

Persuaded, the patient agreed to begin the inpatient treatment. Chuna manual therapy, bee venom therapy, and Motion Style Acupuncture Treatment resulted in much better effects than expected, with the pain redcued by 50% of its initially reported level after just one week.

Mr. Gang, who was originally skeptical about Korean medicine treatments, began to open up and actively participate in the treatment process. As he be-gan to show a more positive attitude towards the treatment, his quadriceps began to regain their strength, allowing him to walk up stairs. He eventually became well enough to receive outpatient care. We continued to provide him with reinforcement treatments, which helped his body recover to a healthy state, in addition to enabling the reabsorption of the ruptured disc. To this day, I am motivated just by thinking about the patient's elated face when his recovery was confirmed through MRI images. Earning the trust of the patient has an important impact on the outcome. I learned that such trust is built not through words, but through the physical improvements of treatment. Friendly attitudes and detailed explanations are important for doctors to incorporate into their practices, but in the end, patients gain trust in their doctors when they see positive developments as a result of treatment. Mr. Gang's case is especially precious to me because it taught me this valuable lesson.

Maintenance Is the Best Disc Treatment

Dr. Seung-cheol Yeom
(Gwangju Jaseng Hospital of Korean Medicine)

There are countless disc patients that I have treated in the past 15 years that have a sad story. Some of the most difficult cases, however, involve patients who were successfully treated but experienced relapses due to bad management of their conditions. It is difficult to experience such extreme pain once, and worse to support someone through it multiple times. This case is included to raise awareness about the importance of post-treatment management for back disc patients.

Mr. Jin-cheol Song (male, age 38) had received inpatient care for back disc herniation at Jaseng back in 2005, before I joined the hospital. I do not know who was in charge of treating him, but it seemed that the treatment results were quite good. Ten years later, however, Mr. Song came to me because his back pain had recurred. Unlike 10 years prior, his pain was so severe that he was not able to walk, sit, or lie down. Quoting the patient, it was a pain that felt as if his "bones would break and his legs would burst."

MRI images showed that his discs were in such bad condition that someone not trained to review MRIs could identify the condition. We immediately began an intensive inpatient care regimen. Because he had been treated at Jaseng 10 years ago, the patient had a good understanding of the procedure. Most of the symptoms were alleviated after 3 weeks of hospitalization.

Mr. Song returned to the hospital four months later. His disc had ruptured again after he indiscriminately engaged in physical activities.

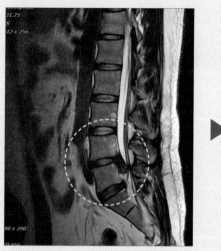
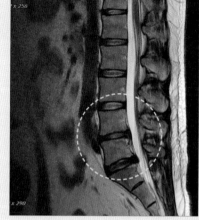

Before treatment

After treatment

Before and after the 1st disc treatment

A ruptured disc was found between the L4 and L5 vertebra. The patient had received Korean medicine treatments, after which the ruptured disc completely reabsorbed.

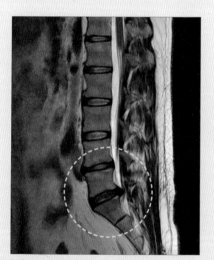

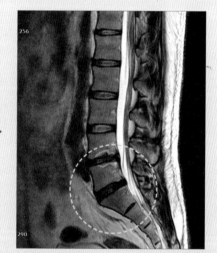

Before treatment

After treatment

Before and after the 2nd disc treatment

Due to poor management, the disc between the L5 and S1 vertebra ruptured amd penetrated the posterior longitudinal ligament. The disc reabsorbed after Korean medicine treatment. The patient is making an effort to manage the condition.

During his previous hospitalization, the disc between the L4 and L5 vertebra had ruptured. MRI images taken this time showed that the previously damaged disc was completely reabsorbed. It was the disc between the L5 and S1 vertebra that had acutely ruptured. During the 71 days of the inpatient treatment program, the patient had to receive more than the equivalent of twelve months of rehabilitation treatments. I used all available methods including Shinbaro herbal medicine, nerve root recovery therapy, and Chuna manual therapy, hoping that the patient's condition would not relapse again.

Because his condition had relapsed twice already due to poor management, Mr. Song had a different attitude this time. Although the treatment period was lengthy and the improvement was slow, the patient continued to manage his mind and body while receiving the treatments. Even when he was not experiencing any symptoms, he regularly returned to my office to continue to manage his condition. We conducted imaging tests to check on his damaged disc and confirmed that the ruptured disc had been completely reabsorbed.

Even when the doctor providing the treatment is highly skilled, without the patient's own effort to maintain his or her health, spinal diseases can recur. I hope that all patients suffering from spinal conditions learn from this case and commit to more focused efforts to help manage their conditions.

Curing A Childhood Friend's Herniated Disc

Dr. Seong-hwan Park
(Jamsil Jaseng Hospital of Korean Medicine)

On a workday filled with emergency patients, I found my phone vibrating with messages from a close friend, Sang-jin Kim (male, age 35). We had been in the same elementary school class, and had been close, frequently hanging out at each other's houses. But because we had both married relatively early and kept busy with our work, we had not kept in contact as often as we had planned. I was happy that my friend had called, but I was also worried that something might have happened. My concerns were confirmed when I picked up the phone: My friend clearly sounded like he was in pain.

"Seong-hwan. You know my back has always been bad... I hurt so much that I can't move... I'm trying to get to your hospital... What do I do?" When I saw my friend at the hospital, he was clearly in pain. I remembered that my friend's back has always been bad and that his older brother had undergone back surgery.

I learned that my friend also had surgery because of a ruptured disc. It was that treated disc that had ruptured again, causing nerve root compression. The discs between L3 and L4, and a second disc between L4 and L5 were protruding. I felt bad for not knowing that my friend's back was in such a bad state.

I came to know that he had been suffering back pain for the past year and had quit his job because of it. Every conventional medicine hospital he had visited recommended surgery, but since the disc that already undergonsurgery were ruptured again, he decided against another operation. That was why he called me.

We immediately began the process of inpatient treatment. I prescribed oral analgesic and painkilling injections. He struggled to stand up and going to the bathroom required much effort. Because of the severe symptoms, my friend had not eaten much for 2 weeks, and had lost about 8 kilograms as a result.

Typically, even the most severe disc herniations improve with a month of intensive treatment. My friend's pain did not subside so easily and because his pain fluctuated significantly, he required treatment in the hospital for almost 50 days. I used Shinbaro herbal medicine, pharmacopuncture, Chuna manual therapy, acupuncture, and cupping treatments, and coordinated with conventional medical staff to ensure that my friend got better. After almost 2 months, my friend was finally able to walk the halls without assistance. At which I thought, "I've got it now!"

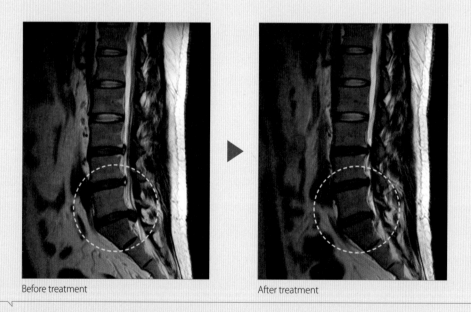

Before treatment

After treatment

Before and after the treatment for a patient who could not even sit up on the bed
The patient was hospitalized for almost 50 days for pain in the right hip, thigh, calf, and ankle. He received outpatient treatments (herbal medicine, pharmacopuncture, Chuna, manual therapies) for 2 months. He is leading a normal life without pain.

After the patient completed his inpatient care period, he transitioned to outpatient care. I administered pharmacopuncture once or twice every week and prescribed regular doses of Shinbaro herbal medicine. Two months after the outpatient care regimen started, my friend felt relief and comfort. The MRI images indicated that the ruptured disc had completely reabsorbed.

My friend started a new job and is now happily working and leading a healthy life. I am thankful to my friend for entrusting me with his health: I am very satisfied that I was able to help my friend through Korean medicine.

Patients with disc conditions like my friend flock to my office. I begin every day at the hospital reminding myself that I heal patients by providing the best treatments, like the ones I gave my friend.

4

Herniated Spinal Discs
Absorb Better

1. Does Pain Subside When Herniated Discs Are Absorbed Back?

Why Do Herniated Discs Cause Pain?

Discs themselves do not have many pain receptors. Pain receptors are primarily located in the nerves posterior to the discs.

In the spinal structure, the discs are located between the vertebral bodies. Elements of the vertebral bones create the spinal cavity, through which a thick nerve bundle passes. This nerve bundle descends through the spinal column. At each spinal level, nerve roots exit in pairs. The discs are located anterior to the nerves. When discs rupture and protrude they compress these nerve roots. The compression of the nerves causes pain.

The pain is expressed in different ways depending on the direction in which the discs rupture and which nerves become compressed.

In general, more pressure is applied to the posterior aspect of a disc. That is why discs rupture posteriorly. In some cases, however, they rupture more anterior. In such cases, not much pain is experienced since there are not any nerves in that location. Such patients do not usually feel the need to seek treatment.

When discs rupture posteriorly and compress the nerve, the patient generally experiences pain. Depending on which nerves are involved, the patient may only experience pain in the back, and/or in the buttocks and legs. Sometimes the pain in the extremity is more pronounced than the pain in

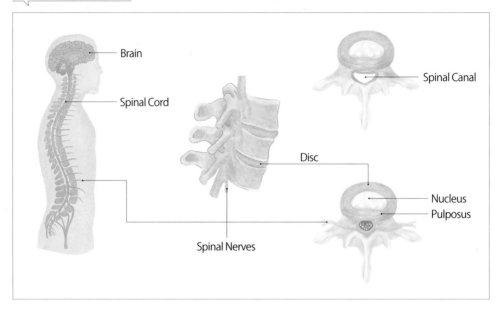

the back. The pain severity is also affected depending on the amount of compression applied to the nerves. If severe, the patient may feel like the corresponding body parts are paralyzed.

30% Absorption of Herniated Discs Reduce Pain

Patients usually feel more pain immediately after a disc ruptures. This is because the membrane that surrounds and protects the disc is damaged as the disc ruptures through it. Inflammation occurs at the site, which inevitably produces pain. The nucleus pulposus stimulates and further inflames the nerves, adding to the pain.

Initial pain will eventually subside – regardless of whether the disc reabsorbs – if the disc is not significantly compressing on a nerve, and the inflammation subsides. In fact, the pain experienced by most disc herniation patients is chemical in nature— the nerves being stimulated by the inflammation. There is less pain associated with the pressure on the nerves.

Even when herniated discs apply significant pressure on nerves, the pain can subside when the discs reabsorb, even just slightly. When that happens, patients who experienced extreme pain soon feel it diminishing.

Even when ruptured discs do not completely reabsorb, pain can completely disappear. According to a 10-year-long study on disc patients conducted by Jaseng, patients feel no pain at the point when30% of the ruptured disc reabsorbs

The time required for ruptured discs to reabsorb varies widely. The process may require from 2 to 12 months. Receiving adequate non-invasive treatments for ruptured discs can shorten the time required for them to reabsorb. Although discs can heal without intervention, non-invasive treatments are recommended to help patients endure the pain, and to reduce the length of time the process would require without intervention.

Self-Diagnosis for Herniated Discs

People who experience back pain will feel worried that their discs might have ruptured. MRI scans are required to accurately diagnose disc herniation, but there are home tests that patients can use.

▶ Lift ing the legs
One of the most commonly known self-diagnosis methods is to lie down on the back and lift the legs. If it is diffi cult to lift the legs or soreness and tingling sensations are felt when the legs are lift ed to about 30 to 60 degrees, back disc herniation should be suspected. Also, if the legs do not lift as well and there is a pain in the shins right below the knees, there is a high chance that discs have been ruptured.

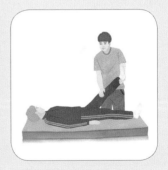

▶ Pushing down the big toes
Lie down flat on the back and move the big toes in the upward direction (toward the head). Then press downward on a big toe, using the opposite foot. If the weak-

ness of the big toe is noted, a nerve is compressed by a
disc in the back.

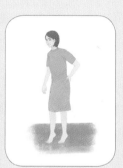

▶ Talking on tiptoes

Walk on tiptoes as if doing ballet dancing. If pain is experienced in the process of taking steps are difficult, there is a
need to conduct more precise disc tests.

▶ Stand straight and walk on heels

Stand upright and walk on heels. If taking steps is diffi cult
or pain is felt in the process, disc herniation may be suspected.

▶ Sit on the fl oor with legs stretched out and bend the torso towards the front

Sit on the fl oor with legs stretched out forward, and then
stretch the hands towards the feet to bend the torso slowly. Cough a couple of times when the torso is bent as much
as possible. If severe pain is felt in the back, there is a high
chance that herniation is present in the back discs.

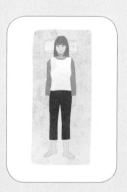

▶ Measure the length of the legs

Measuring the length of the legs is not directly to check
the status of the discs. Th is is to see if the spine and the
hip are structured properly, which is a factor contributes
to the risk of disc herniation. Measure the length of both
legs while lying down fl at on the back. If one of the legs is
shorter, the hip is distorted or the spine is unstable. Since it
is diffi cult to accurately measure the leg lengths if the legs
are intentionally skewed or the person has a bad posture,
the measurement must be taken while lying down fl at on
the back.

Another way to do this is to measure the legs while lying down on the stomach. Th
e patient lies down on the stomach and then bends the knees, and another person
compares the height of the raised ankles. If one of the legs is shorter, this means that
the hip is distorted or the spine is unstable.

2. More Disc Ruptures Mean Better Absorption

Herniated Discs Absorb Back Even Without Surgery

Herniated discs absorb with adequate non-invasive treatments, even without surgery. In fact, if the patient can endure the pain, the ruptured discs will absorb naturally if left alone. When the nucleus pulposus leaks from a ruptured disc, the macrophages absorb the leaking liquid. Even if only 30% of the ruptured disc is absorbed back, the pain will dissipate completely.

Jaseng Spine and Joint Research Institute conducted a study on patients who were diagnosed with disc herniation that received integrative Korean medicine treatment at the 19 Jaseng locations from February 2012 to December 2015. Patients whose discs were expected to absorb were observed for any progression of their disease.

Among the 505 patients that met the criteria for the study, 54.2% were initially recommended surgery at another hospital when their discs first ruptured. Most of the subjects received non-invasive treatments. The average age of the patients was approximately 39 years old, and 60% of the subjects were men. Of the patients enrolled in the study 53.3% had disc herniations between L4 and L5, and 38.8% had ruptured discs between L5 and S1.

MRI images were obtained before and after receiving treatment. The scans demonstrated that the ruptured discs had not reabsorbed after treatment in only 19 patients. In the remaining 486 patients, the ruptured discs had reabsorbed, and 220 patients had experienced more than a 50% reduction in the size of their ruptured discs.

Among the 505 patients, 186 (38.6%) were admitted to the hospital to receive treatment, and the remainder received integrative Korean medicine treatments on an outpatient basis. The average inpatient care period was approximately 34 days while the average outpatient care period was 33 days. The average length of treatment period, including both inpatient and outpatient care, was around 45 days. Most of the patients were prescribed herbal medicine (96.4%), acupuncture (96.4%), and Chuna manual therapy (87.9%). Some patients received bee venom therapy (65.0%), pharmacopuncture (53.3%), electroacupuncture (46.5%), and cupping treatments (22.6%).

The progress of these patients proved quite impressive as well. The patients were tracked for 50 months after the study and 68.4% did not experience any back pain during the tracking period, with more than 90% of the patients expressing satisfaction for the Korean medicine treatments they had received. The results of this large-scale disc absorption study were published in an international academic journal in 2017 and were reported by major Korean media outlets.

More Acute and More Ruptures Mean Better Absorption

Although the degree of disc rupture and pain level are not always proportional, generally a larger disc rupture results in more severe pain. In addition, patients whose discs rupture suddenly, as opposed to gradually, tend to experience more pain.

The more severe the pain, the greater the patients' anxiety about the condition. When severe pain prevents walking and moving, it is inevitable for patients to want to seek surgery immediately. Ironically, more acute and more severe disc ruptures tend to indicate that the damaged discs will actually reabsorb better.

Research suggests that larger ruptures lead to better disc reabsorption. That is cases in which the weakened annulus fibrosus only allows slight extrusion of nucleus pulposus, l reabsorb more quickly than cases in which the annulus fibrosus s significantly disrupted allowing larger amounts of the nucleus pulposus to extrude.

More damage to the annulus fibrosus and the posterior longitudinal ligament result in greater amounts of nucleus pulposus leaking into the epidural space. The epidural space is where the nerves branch out from the spinal cord. When discs enter this space, the immune system recognizes the material as foreign and macrophages are activated.

In a study conducted in 2012, Tamer Orief reported that larger extrusions tend to better reabsorb. He believed that this occurs because larger ruptured disc fragments have more moisture. The additional moisture means that dehydration takes place more readily, which in turn increases inflammatory responses. The macrophages consume the extruded discs more quickly, leading to faster reabsorption.

A study on ruptured disc reabsorption conducted by Jaseng should be understood in the same context. Jaseng Hospital of Korean Medicine published the findings of cases involving patients who received Korean medicine non-invasive treatments that experienced pain alleviation and ruptured disc reabsorption. The study published in an international academic journal included the more cases than previous studies on ruptured disc reabsorption.

This study measured the volume of ruptured disc material before and after treatment. More severely damaged discs tended to reabsorb faster after treatment. Also, on average, more than half of the volume of these extruded discs reabsorbed, leading to

Reabsorption process of ruptured discs

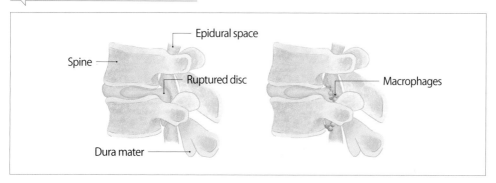

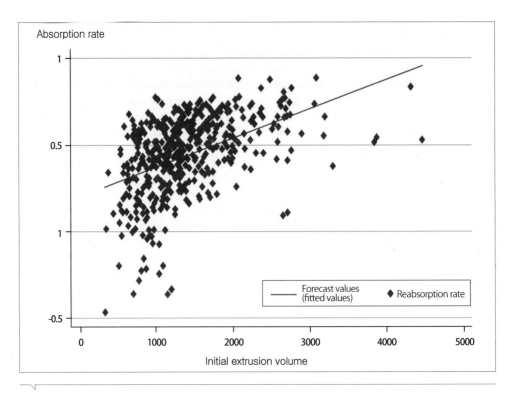

Correlation between the initial extrusion volume and reabsorption rate. A reabsorption rate of 1 means 100% reabsorption, and 0.5 means 50% reabsorption.

complete resolution of pain. The reduction in pain was noted even before the ruptured disc reabsorption could be confirmed through MRI images.

Can the Reabsorption of Herniated Discs Be Predicted?

When discs rupture, they can reabsorb without surgery. This reabsorption process is generally faster and more complete for larger and more acute ruptures. Do all ruptured discs reabsorb back without surgery? No, that is not the case. According to observations of disc patients at Jaseng Hospital for over a decade, 70% of such patients had their ruptured discs reabsorbed.

What about pain? Back and leg pain, the most typical symptoms of disc herniation, completely disappeared in patients whose ruptured discs reabsorbed more than 30%. Even in patients whose ruptured discs did not absorb, 67% reported significant pain alleviation. Only a small number of remaining patients absolutely required surgery.

Doctors who treat disc herniations would like to be able to know which patients will have their ruptured discs reabsorb and which ones will not. Accurate prediction of ruptured disc reabsorption could eliminate the need for unnecessary surgery, as well as knowing which patients would not benefit from non-invasive treatments.

According to a Finnish researcher, neovascular distribution, a barometer of ruptured disc absorption, can be measured using MRI contrast-enhanced testing. This method involves injecting a fluorescent contrast medium before conducting MRI scans. If the contrast medium reveals increased neovascularization around the damaged discs, there is a greater likelihood of faster and more complete disc absorption. The risks of contrast medium injection must always take into account the possibility of serious side effects.

Although inflammation around the ruptured discs causes pain, it ironically activates the macrophages, which result in ruptured disc absorption. As such, inhibiting the inflammatory responses may interfere with the disc absorption process. One researcher studied the use of steroid injections intended to block the inflammatory mechanism, and found that the method can impede ruptured disc absorption. Due to the small number of clinical case studies at this time, a definitive conclusion is not possible at the given moment.

Age, damage to the annulus fibrosus and posterior longitudinal ligaments, and many other factors impact the absorption of ruptured discs. Additional research is needed to provide a more accurate prediction of ruptured disc absorption. Jaseng Spine and Joint Research Institute is studying more than 1,000 disc extrusion patients to develop a program that will predict the absorption of ruptured discs. The development of this program is expected to make it easier to determine the best treatment options for disc herniation patients.

3. Disc Absorption Does Not Restore the Spine to Its Original State

Spinal Discs Change Constantly

Jaseng Hospital of Korean Medicine conducted a study of 128 disc herniation patients, tracking the progress of their diseases for 5 years with annual MRI scans.

The results of the scans reveal that spinal discs change their shape and condition every year. In some years they were protruded, while in other years, they were not.

Ruptured disc absorption refers to the process in which the extruded nucleus pulposus naturally decomposes and is absorbed back into the body.

The mechanism is similar to how other lesions and injuries naturally heal and disappear. While some patients believe that the leaked nucleus pulposus flows back into the disc this is not the case. When discs reabsorb, their size decreases but they do not return to their original state.

Absorbed discs can rupture again. Of note, previously ruptured discs lose moisture and become firmer. Discs function better when sufficiently hydrated and supple. When discs become firmer, they are more prone to rerupture.

Patients should be informed of this possibility.

Changes in Spinal Discs and Pain Do Not Always Go Together

Although disc shapes are constantly changing, most people are not aware of these fluctuations. This was observed in a study involving 128 patients. Some patients actually experienced more pain when previously protruded discs became smaller while others do not appreciate a change in pain even when the protrusion became worse.

Disc treatment is more complicated than pain treatment. As noted by research, disc conditions can worsen in the absence of pain. Patients need to be advised to pay close attention to their conditions regardless of pain. In addition, since individual patients experience different processes of disc rupture, absorption, extrusion, and reabsorption. Patients need a primary doctor who can manage the treatment process over time. Ongoing communication between patients and doctors is important in the management of disc related pain.

4. Different Treatments and Management Strategies Are Needed for Different Stages of Herniated Disc

Disc Herniation Occurs in Stages

Although disc herniations often occur in stages, this is not true in all cases. Discs sometimes rupture so abruptly that the nucleus pulposus suddenly is released into surrounding tissue. In most cases however, discs gradually rupture over time. Phases of disc herniation can be divided into 4 stages depending on the severity of the rupture.

Stage 1 involves a slight swelling of the disc, which is called the bulging stage.

Although the nucleus pulposus is swollen due to a weakened annulus fibrosus, the nerves are not contacted or compressed. In this stage, pain if it exists is not too severe and is mostly isolated to the back.

Stage 2 involves the swollen nucleus pulposus pushing through the annulus fibrosus. This is called the protrusion stage. If the disc compresses a nerve, the patient will experience pain that they often feel in a leg in addition to the back pain.

In stage 3, the weakened annulus fibrosus has more difficulty maintaining the nucleus pulposus. As the nucleus pulposus escapes through the annulus fibrosus, extrusion occurs. As in the case of protrusion, the pain in this stage is felt in both the back and leg(s).

In stage 4, the nucleus pulposus that extruded through the annulus fibro-

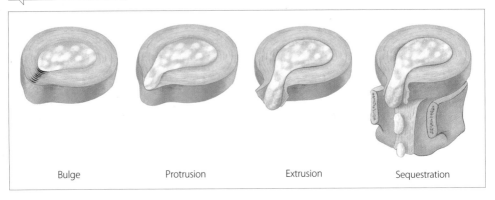

Bulge Protrusion Extrusion Sequestration

sus separates from the disc. This is called sequestration.

Pain Is No Sure Indicator in Early Stages of Herniated Discs

The term early stages do not necessarily refer to only bulging or protruding discs with milder herniation. "Early stages" refers to when the patient first experiences the pain, regardless of the actual degree of the disc herniation. Some patients will have felt back pain for the very first time when they visit the hospital, only to find that their discs have severely ruptured as the degree of herniation and pain are not always proportional.

Treatment approaches and management methods should be different for patients in their early stages than those in their chronic stages. In early stages, patients are often in more severe pain because they are more sensitive to back pain.

Patients with back pain frequently request surgery, probably because they desire to escape from such severe pain as quickly as possible. Some patients choose surgery because they are alarmed by the severe pain they have never felt before or because the pain has returned or worsened.

Since pain can instill significant fear and anxiety in disc herniation patients, medical professionals focus on treating the pain in the early stages of the disease. It is not very difficult to alleviate the pain earlier in the process. Even the most severe pain can be significantly reduced with non-invasive treatment. Motion Style Acupuncture Treatment and Chuna manual therapy can eliminate the pain within a matter of days. Many patients arrive at our hospital on a stretcher but walk back home after 2 to 3 days of treatment.

Patients should not let their guard down because they are no longer feeling pain. Ligaments and cartilages recover at a rate independent of the experienced pain levels. Patients need to be reminded of this fact.

While pain can subside within days, it takes time for the ligaments and muscles surrounding the damaged area to recover. Since the regeneration process takes at least 3 months, patients need to rest sufficiently during the early stages of their disease, taking care not to further damage their discs.

There is one mistake often made by patients who have received non-invasive treatment for their ruptured discs. In treating disc patients in their early stages, doctors emphasize that they need to address and correct the habits that places stress on the discs. When the pain subsides, however, patients forget the doctor's instructions and resume the bad habits that caused the condition in the first place.

The lack of pain does not mean that the cause of disc herniation has disappeared. Even when the ruptured discs are absorbed, inflammation has disappeared, and the pain has gone, the annulus fibrosus has changed. If the patient continues the habits that places stress on the back, the previously damaged discs can rupture again at anytime.

Chronic Disc Herniation Requires Patience and Relaxation

If adequate treatments are not provided and bad habits are not corrected during the early stages of disc herniation, the condition can become chronic. Chronic disc herniation has symptoms similar to degenerative disc herniation: Mild pain can be intermittent. During this repeated ebb and flow of pain, the discs become weaker and more damaged.

Most chronic back pain is caused by degenerative changes. As one ages, the discs that were once soft and elastic become firmer and thinner. The thinner and firmer discs cannot absorb shock as well and the shape of vertebral bones changes, resulting in bony structures that can further exacerbate the disc conditions.

The problem is that most patients ignore the pain, missing an opportunity to stop the progression of the disease. Further, their fear of surgery or the consequences of surgery causes patients to avoid seeking an accurate diagnosis or to solely depend on folk therapies. Such patients come to the hospital only after their condition has worsened significantly.

In fact, not many patients come to the hospital in the early stages of disc herniation. Most of them see a doctor when the condition has become chronic. Of course, chronic disc herniation is more difficult to treat, but some patients experience dramatic improvements despite the chronic nature of their condition. Doctors feel satisfied when their treatments allow chronic disc patients to improve.

When treating chronic disc patients, about 90% of them gradually improve within about 3 months. The remaining 10% do not show any signs of improvement for the first 3 months, followed by significant improvement usually towards the beginning of the 6th month.

It is difficult to determine the treatment period for such patients who show gradual progress. There are no fixed solutions for them.

Since the treatment direction must be determined based on the doctor's experience, chronic disc patients are advised to seek help from more experienced specialists.

Chronic disc patients recover at different rates. The ability to recover and adapt is different for each individual, which means that the speed of recovery will vary. Some patients adapt within 2 months, while the process can take more than 6 months for others. Although the recovery speed can differ from individual to individual, with persistent treatment, all patients will reach a point of recovery. Patients with more chronic problems will not react much to the treatment initially, recovering slowly nevertheless through the human body's power of self-healing.

Since the recovery rates for chronic disc conditions differ, patients and their doctors must communicate effectively. In order to prevent the patient from becoming anxious and to ensure the effectiveness of the treatment, the doctor must consistently explain to the patient the symptoms and outcomes of the disease.

Jaseng doctors do sometimes recommend surgery over non-invasive treatment depending on the responses of chronic disc patients. Doctors often feel lost if their patients do not respond well to more than 3 months of treatment. New doctors are especially quick to abandon non-invasive treatment and recommend surgery because they have not been exposed to many different chronic disc patients.

However, as previously addressed if the patient has not recovered yet, it is only because the patient's body is not ready for recovery.

In some cases, patients will insist on continuing non-invasive treatment, and finally recover after 5 to 6 months of treatment.

Many chronic disc patients will not respond quickly to non-invasive treatment. Patients are advised to remember this and to remain calm; they should communicate with their doctors about even the smallest things that could impact the recovery and the conditions of their discs.

One of the hidden truths about the lengthy recovery process of many chronic disc patients is that their bodies are already severely damaged from painkillers and injections, even before they begin Korean medicine treatments. Steroid analgesics used on patients to reduce their pain does not rid the body of the symptoms; they merely suppress the symptoms.

When pain is present, people instinctively take action to address their condition. However, when pain is removed by administering potent analgesics, patients often take no precaution and continue the bad habits that placed stress on the discs As such, in order for chronic disc patients to properly benefit from non-invasive treatments, they should stop taking the analgesics and learn to endure the pain. If their pain is too great to endure, patients should rest or maintain postures that can reduce the pain to prevent exacerbating the damage on the discs. Patients must participate in treatment and manage their conditions with a more relaxed attitude.

Disc patients must understand that their treatment program is a long journey, and that they need to maintain an attitude of positivity and endurance by thinking that they will get better with treatment, however long it may take. Chronic disc herniation can take a long time to address, but it is rarely incurable. Most patients will see improvement if they patiently continue to receive Korean medicine non-invasive treatments.

5. Inpatient Care Can Help Treat Herniated Discs

Inpatient Care Is Not Just for Surgery

Most patients who are admitted to the hospital are scheduled for surgery. There are not many countries in the world in which hospitals admit patients who do not need surgery. Even in countries with advanced medical systems like the U.S., patients are admitted for only 3 to 4 days for surgery. Jaseng Hospital of Korean Medicine, however, often provides inpatient care for patients who are receiving noninvasive treatments. They are hospitalized for 2 to 3 weeks to receive non-invasive treatments and practice a systematic rehabilitation exercise regimen.

Why does Jaseng provide intensive inpatient treatment programs accompanied by an exercise rehabilitation program coupled with rest? The goal of such practice is to help patients personally experience the treatability of chronic disc conditions through inpatient care programs.

If patients were not satisfied with the inpatient treatment programs offered by Jaseng, our inpatient wards would be empty. On the contrary, our beds are always filled with patients. Even though the treatments are not inexpensive, our patients note the value of our inpatient care programs.

Inpatient Care Has Different Values for Acute and Chronic Herniated Disc Conditions

The value of inpatient care for patients is different for acute and chronic back conditions. Acute disc herniation patients choose to undergo surgery because they cannot engage in daily activities due to severe pain. In such cases, hospitalizing the patient to provide pain-relieving treatments can provide immediate help. Although 3 weeks of inpatient care cannot completely treat the disease, providing such prompt relief can prevent the patient from choosing surgery.

Also, learning more about disc herniation during their hospitalization period often encourages patients to take better care of their discs even after they are discharged.

Inpatient care also prevents acute disc herniation from progressing to a chronic condition. Even with highly responsive treatments, 5 to 10% of back pain eventually becomes a chronic condition. To prevent this, the symptoms must be treated intensively at the beginning. Patients whose disc herniation is expected to become chronic should be given more intensive pain remedies in addition to treatments directed at the surrounding muscles and ligaments. This can decrease the probability that the condition will become chronic. This is the value that acute disc herniation patients can expect from seeking inpatient care.

Chronic patients should consider inpatient care, as such a program can help them develop hope and confidence that their discs will fully recover. Chronic disc patients are often accustomed to pain because they have been suffering for extended periods of time. They also do not actively seek treatment because their pain does not usually render them immobile and because they do not believe that any treatment will help them.

It is of note that many patients have already invested considerable amounts of time and money into treating their conditions, and falsely believe they have become "experts" in disc herniation.

In many cases, chronic disc patients who receive outpatient care do not experience as quick of a recovery as acute disc patients. Many of them do not initially respond well to outpatient treatments. This encourages them to change hospitals only after a couple of months of treatment.

Inpatient care is different. Chronic patients who receive 3 weeks of intensive inpatient care will experience satisfactory levels of pain reduction, allowing them to feel that their condition is improving. That is, the value of inpatient care for chronic patients lies in the fact that it gives them hope that they will get better. Inpatient care not only provides treatment but also provides an escape from the habits and environment that were the root causes of chronic pain. This will encourage the admitted chronic patient even more.

The hospitalization period provides an opportunity to reflect on their bad lifestyle habits and realize that they can recover from their disc conditions. This strongly motivates them to actively participate in the treatment process.

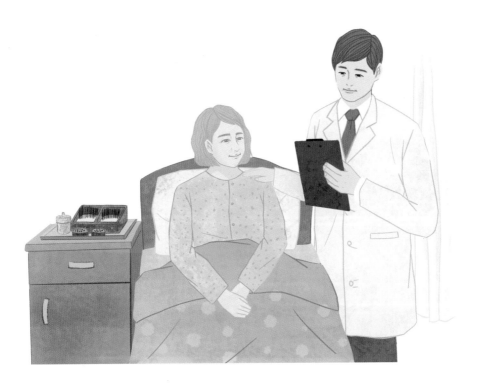

———

5

Surgery Must Be
the Final Resort

1. Failed Back Surgery Syndrome (FBSS) Is Worse Than Herniated Discs

People Who Suffered More After Surgery

Ms. Yeong-ja Gwon (female, age 63) had been suffering from a back disc for about a decade and underwent an operation where 4 screws were placed into her spine in 2000. Because she had been suffering from back conditions since her mid-30s, Ms. Gwon had been receiving physical therapy from a university hospital since 1989 to manage her pain. Because of the chronic nature of her pain, she had been enduring even severe pain as a normal part of her life.

Her life went on like that for a more than ten years, until 2000. That year, her pain became unbearable. Even when she simply sat down in the driver's seat, her pain became so severe that she could not breathe. Although she was scared of surgery, Ms. Gwon agreed to undergo surgery, believing that the operation would free her from chronic back pain. The results, however, were disappointing.

Her pain worsened after the surgery, and for the first 5 months after the operation, she was not able to ambulate on her own. She needed the assistance of her family members just to go to the bathroom, and she had to crawl on her arms and legs to get around inside her house.

Desperate, she returned to the hospital. The answer that Ms. Gwon received was that although the surgery went well, the regions surrounding the operated area had become worse. Ms. Gwon was disappointed with this news. The constant back and leg pains were torture enough, but she was also conflicted by the fact that she could not survive even a day without the constant help of someone else.

After suffering for 2 years, another surgery was recommended for Ms. Gwon. Because she had such a painful experience following her first surgery, she inquired after a hospital that could treat her condition without surgery, and arrived at the doorstep of Jaseng Hospital of Korean Medicine. Because she had tried almost everything to cure her back condition during the past 2 years, Ms. Gwon first agreed to take Shinbaro herbal medicine and receive Chuna manual therapy, without high expectations. The extreme back pain that had pestered the patient for such a long time, however, dissipated within a few months of beginning the treatments, returning her mind and body to a normal state.

Mr. Sang-wu Choi (male, age 38) also suffered greatly after undergoing back surgery for his disc problems, like Ms. Gwon. The operation on his back took place in March 2004. When he began suffering symptoms such as severe back pain, leg weakness, and paralysis in the lower half of his body, he became scared and ended up undergoing surgery within a week. He did not question the process.

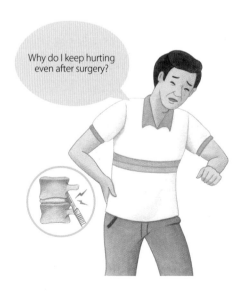

He did not have much knowledge about the surgery, but he was overly reassured by the hospital's promise that he could be discharged within 3 days of surgery.

He said, "They said it would be okay. That I would be discharged in 3 days. That's why I thought that disc herniation was a disease as mild as a boil."

The surgery, however, did not meet his expectations. His pain did not subside even after the surgery, and he could not endure the pain without painkillers and muscle relaxants. Moreover, about 8 months after the surgery, the disc herniation relapsed. He could not sit or stand because of extreme back pain. Even though he had originally not even considered surgery, all of the hospitals he visited recommended artificial disc placement.

Mr. Choi, wanting to avoid an artificial disc surgery, came to Jaseng Hospital of Korean Medicine as a last resort. Examinations revealed that his discs were severely ruptured and were blocking off four-fifths of the nerves. Because his spine was distorted, his legs were noticeably unequal in length. Fortunately, he was able to walk without pain after 50 days of Chuna manual therapy, Motion Style Acupuncture Treatment, bee venom therapy, and Shinbaro herbal medicine.

There are people who, like Ms. Gwon and Mr. Choi, experience even more pain after disc surgery. There must be nothing more disheartening than having one's condition worsen after surgery. Of course, not all patients who undergo surgery face such negative results, but even the smallest possibility should not be risked.

Surgery is not a panacea. It does not guarantee that herniated discs will recover. Decisions to receive surgery must be made with deliberation and caution. Though many patients choose to undergo surgery because they want their pain to go away as quickly as possible, rushing to a decision can lead to disastrous results. The average life expectancy has risen to close to 100 years. Longevity, however, is not always something to be celebrated. There are many requirements for someone who wishes to live to be 100, but the most important is good health. Having to rely on the assistance of others while suffering from terrible pain until the age of 100 is not a blessing; it is closer to misfortune.

Patients who have suffered from the consequences of disc surgery know the agony of living with chronic pain. Numerous patients continue to experience pain and even worsen after surgery. There is a reason that failed back surgery syndrome has become such a prominent phenomenon.

Failed Back Surgery Syndrome Destroys Quality of Life

Failed back surgery syndrome became an official term in the field of physiological science when it was first mentioned on Pub Med, one of the most renowned medical science journal websites in the U.S. The term itself is chilling. That is why Korean doctors are not fond of this term. Korean doctors argue that the term "failed back surgery syndrome" creates the misconception that these symptoms are caused by back surgery failures. These doctors are working to change the term to "post-back surgery pain syndrome."

The important thing is not the term, however. It is the reality of effects and consequences of such surgery. Regardless of whether the word "failure" is used, the important thing is that there are patients whose conditions have worsened after disc surgery. More than anything, many such patients experience sharp decreases in quality of life that can cause them to develop depression or even their will to live.

Failed back surgery syndrome became a global issue when the journal PAIN published a study about quality of life in regards to pain in 2010.

This study examined 25 papers to investigate the level of happiness that patients with various diseases reported to have experienced.

This research encompassed information about pains caused by diabetes, failed surgery, cancer, heart failures, stroke, and most other severe diseases, to understand the patients' qualities of life.

A value of 1 indicated the highest possible level of happiness and quality of life, and a value of 0 indicated the lowest possible level of happiness and quality of life.

The study concluded that failed back surgery syndrome is more painful than cancer, stroke, or diabetes. Compared to the fact that the average perceived quality of life for cancer and stroke patients ranged from 0.3 to 0.4, that of failed back surgery syndrome

Quality of life comparison for different types of diseases

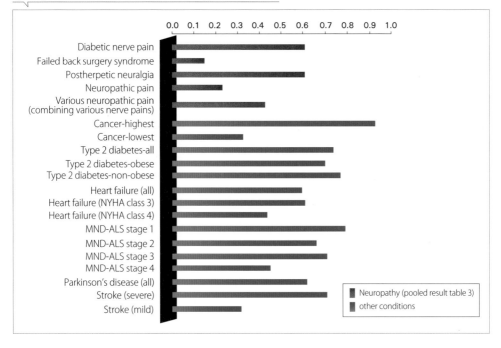

patients was less than half those values, at 0.12.

Failed back surgery syndrome is defined as a state in which one or more back surgeries does not improve the condition, worsening the symptoms or triggering relapse.

Patients begin suffering from this syndrome at different points after back surgery. In some cases, it appears 3 months after surgery, while in others, it takes up to a year.

In fact, it is not very important when symptoms return after surgery. Few people opt to have back surgery to enjoy relief for only a few years. When one chooses to undergo surgery, they make this difficult decision hoping that surgery will not be needed again. However, patients should remember that it is much more difficult than expected for that hope to be fulfilled.

Integrative Korean medicine Treatment Is Effective Against Failed Back Surgery Syndrome

The term "failed back surgery syndrome" may cause people to think that it is the result of back surgery gone wrong. However, the syndrome is caused even when the surgery is successful; ligament damage, spine structure change, and other factors can make the pain continue even after surgery. In sum, failed back surgery syndrome does not necessarily occur because of a "failed surgery."

In general, 15% of patients who undergo spine surgery are known to suffer from this syndrome, which is difficult to treat. Although different types of treatments have been tested and studied, most patients typically only see around a 10% to 20% improvement in terms of pain relief.

In comparison, integrative Korean medicine treatments are very effective. Jaseng Spine and Joint Research Institute provided 16 weeks of integrative Korean medicine treatment to 120 patients suffering from failed back surgery syndrome and tracked their progress for 1 year. The patients were examined at 24 weeks and 1 year after the treatment program was completed. There was improvement in 89.4% of the subjects after 24 weeks, and 79.2% provided the same answer after a year.

To conduct the study, the research team selected adult men and women between the ages of 18 and 60 who had received back surgery between November of 2011 and September of 2014. The patients had experienced back or lower extremity pain sometime during the three weeks prior to the study, or had had their symptoms return within a year after receiving surgery. The subjects reported pain scores (VAS, visual analog scale) of 6 or higher. The patients were prescribed a 16-week treatment program involving Shinbaro herbal medicine, Shinbaro pharmacopuncture, Chuna manual therapy, and Motion Style Acupuncture Treatment. To ensure the accuracy of the program's effectiveness, the patients were recommended to not receive other back pain treatments. 24 weeks after the program, the patients were interviewed in person. One year after the program, they were interviewed via phone about their physical conditions.

The in-person interviews conducted after 24 weeks revealed that the patients' back and leg pain index scores (VAS), disability index scores (ODI), and health level index scores (SF-36) had improved drastically following the treatments. The phone interviews conducted after 1 year also revealed that the patients had maintained healthy conditions, in terms of pain and disability. Comparing values between the first in-person interview and the second phone interview, the average overall pain score increased from 2.9 to 3.3, but the average leg pain score fell from 2.4 to 1.7. The disability index measures the ability to perform 10 daily activities, including sitting, standing, walking, and carrying objects. This average score improved in the 1-year interview compared to that reported in the 24-week interview.

In response to a question about their current health conditions during the phone interview, the patients reported that their average health level measurement score had improved from 42.8 to 62.7.

As shown in the research study, integrative Korean medicine treatment yielded positive results in terms of pain, disability, and quality of life. Furthermore, the effects lasted at least 1 year after the treatments, leading to the conclusion that it is the most ef-

Before and 24 weeks after integrative Korean medicine treatments were provided to failed back surgery syndrome patients

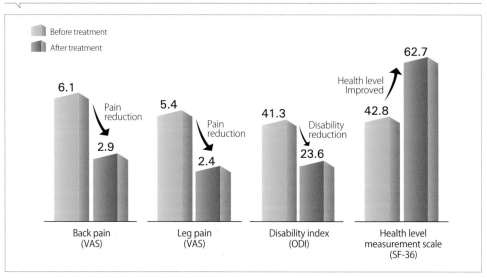

fective treatment for failed back surgery syndrome currently in existence. Because failed back surgery syndrome is so difficult to treat, only 10 to 20% of patients see improvement even after receiving integrated conventional medicine treatments (which include painkillers, physical therapy, and injections). As such, many patients undergo surgery, in which an electric stimulator is inserted on to the spinal cord. Even this procedure can only be considered successful with over 50% improvement of reported pain levels. Since Jaseng's integrative Korean medicine treatments had over 50% improvement on average without surgery, these results are quite encouraging. The study was published in Plos One, the official journal of the U.S. Public Library of Science.

2. Only a Small Number of Patients Actually Require Surgery

Only 5–10% of All Patients Require Surgery

Although opinions vary among scholars, only about 5 to 10% of all disc patients truly require surgery due to severe nerve damage. Campbell's "Orthopedics," considered the textbook of orthopedics, claims that only 2% of all back pain patients need to undergo surgery. This aligns with the idea that 90 to 95% of all disc patients can be completely healed with non-invasive treatments alone.

Jaseng Hospital of Korean Medicine has been conducting clinical studies to confirm if such theoretical findings correlate with the practices of Jaseng non-invasive treatments. Jaseng Hospital of Korean Medicine worked with the University of North Carolina research team to study 128 lumbar disc herniation patients for 6 months while providing weekly treatments involving Shinbaro herbal medicine, acupuncture, bee venom therapy, and Chuna manual therapy.

The results showed that 95% of all patients saw significant improvements in their symptoms to the point where they could perform everyday activities, proving the theoretical findings discussed above. Some of the 128 patients had surgery recommended. In the same group, 94% experienced significant pain relief.

As demonstrated, 95% of disc patients can be fully healed without surgery. Thus, patients are advised to decide whether to undergo surgery only after carefully considering if they are among the 5 to 10% truly requiring an operation.

The 4 Criteria for Surgery

Surgery must be the last resort for patients when ruptured discs cannot be improved with non-invasive treatments. Although most disc conditions can be treated with non-invasive treatments, surgery is required in some cases. When a patient's disc is severely ruptured with extreme nerve damage, causing extensive pain and paralytic symptoms, surgery is required. The following criteria can be used to consider whether a patient needs surgery.

The first condition is the impairment of rectal or bladder functions. When ruptured discs compress the nerves innervating the bladder, patients will suffer from urination and bowel movement issues. Called cauda equina syndrome, these symptoms involve a gradual loss of rectal or bladder function. Since such cases are emergencies, patients are advised to undergo surgery emergently.

Second, parasthesias or anesthesia in the groin or anal regions are symptoms of cauda equina syndrome. Patients in this category must pay close attention to their conditions.

The third case is one in which motor muscle strength worsens progressively. If the patient's leg muscle weakness continues to worsen or muscle contractions occur despite non-invasive treatments, and loss of the Achilles tendon reflex is also observed, the patient requires surgery. Since nerves may have been permanently damaged in the case of severe progressive paralysis, these patients must receive surgery as soon as possible to give the affected nerves a chance to heal.

Whether or not surgery is required for non-progressive conditions is a controversial topic. A recent study followed disc rupture patients with muscle strength loss for 1 year; one group received surgery and the other group did not. There were not too many differences between the conditions of the two groups. This indicates that a simple loss of muscle strength does not require surgery. However, if the patient is experiencing progressive loss of muscle strength during treatment, they will likely require surgery. In such cases, the specialist's decision is more important than the patient's judgment.

The fourth condition is one in which non-invasive treatments are not effective or worsen the pain. Some patients experience no improvement or even worsening of the pain despite various non-invasive treatments. In general, acute disc herniation patients who do not experience improvement after 3 months of treatment may require surgery.

3. OX Quiz on Whether Conditions Require Surgery

When Doctors Recommend Surgery

In general, when a doctor states that they "recommend surgery" to a disc patient, the recommendation might not be made out of necessity, but rather because surgery is a quick and simple treatment. As seen in many previous cases, insufficient surgery can inflict critical damage to the discs. As such, patients are advised to exercise caution when a doctor recommends surgery.

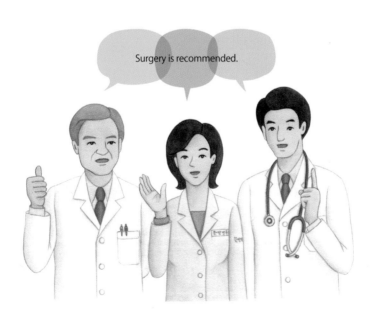

Surgery is recommended.

The best option is to seek a second opinion when a doctor recommends surgery. If at least 3 doctors say that surgery is absolutely necessary, the patient should consider surgery. One of the 3 doctors should be a Korean medicine doctor or a doctor who specializes in non-invasive treatments.

This is because spine and joint doctors have different specialties, including orthopedics, neurosurgery, rehabilitation, and Korean medicine. Depending on their specialty, doctors may wish to take different approaches to treatment.

For example, if the doctor specializes in orthopedics or neurosurgery, he or she may want to provide surgical treatment because that is how they were trained. Korean medicine doctors, on the other hand, will want to recommend Korean medicine treatment. Rather than focusing on the specialty of the doctors, it is more important to treat disc herniation with safer methods. If 3 or more doctors of different specialties recommend surgery for disc herniation, it is likely that the patient requires surgery.

Answer: X

What If the Herniated Nucleus Pulposus Is Compressing the Nerves?

If nucleus pulposus leaks out of ruptured discs, it will absorb better than when the disc is simply protruding. Since patients may recover quickly due to the faster absorption rate, patients should wait until the naturally ruptured disc is absorbed back into the body.

In the past, doctors tried to conduct surgery as soon as possible because they thought the ruptured disc would continue compressing the nerves. Today, however, the general opinion of the medical community is that ruptured discs can reabsorb and disappear with good treatment, which means that surgery is not required. Since non-invasive methods are sufficient in treating ruptured disc or leaking nucleus pulposus, not all patients need to undergo surgery.

Answer: X

What If You Have Herniated Discs, Stenosis, and Degenerative Conditions?

People with bad spine conditions not only have ruptured discs, but may also experience stenosis and degenerative changes. In such cases, surgery should not be performed. Because stenosis or degenerative disc conditions require a more extensive surgery, the operation may put an excessive burden on the spine. Stenosis or degenerative disc conditions not only affect one vertebra, but multiple vertebrae.

When one or two vertebral bodies undergo surgery and are fixed with pedicle screws, the adjacent discs may rupture or degenerate. Spinal vertebrae distribute the body's weight by moving independently of each other. If they are fixed to each other, the bones above and below the fused bones must move more, weakening or degenerating the adjacent discs even further. Although the vertebra may improve, such surgery may cause serious side effects in adjacent segments and organs. As such, patients with severe stenosis and degenerative disc disease are advised not to undergo surgery.

Answer: X

What If the Pain Continues Even After Multiple Back Injections?

Disc patients tend to favor back injections as their preferred treatment. They are, however, not the only way to alleviate back pain. In conventional medicine, patients who have spinal injections are eventually referred for surgery.

Most spinal injections contain steroids, which serve as strong painkilling substances. The pharmaceutical substances used in injection treatments do not strengthen the weakened back, ligaments, and muscles nor recover the damaged nerves. Rather, substances like steroids or lidocaine anesthetize the affected areas.

When the body is anesthetized, the patient will feel less pain, but will have been provided with no fundamental treatment.

Other patients may mistake the reduced pain as a sign that the disease itself has been cured, and return to the harmful lifestyle that caused the disc disease in the first place. When their back pain returns, they again try to solve the problem with injections.

The body gradually builds up resistance to all drugs. Frequent spinal injections will cause the body to build resistance to the administered drugs, reducing the return and duration of effectiveness. If the effects of the drug lasted for 6 months following initial treatment, the duration may decrease to 3 months after continued administration. This period can be reduced down to a week. Because of the body's gradual resistance to and tolerance for the drugs, doctors may end up recommending surgery to their patients.

Even when patients develop resistance to such pharmacological treatments, non-invasive treatments can still enable recovery. Such patients may have a slower recovery than others who have not been exposed to back injections. This is because spinal injections further weaken and damage discs.

Pain is a signal given by the body that indicates there is a problem. If injections eliminate such signals from the body without treating it, the ruptured discs will inevitably worsen.

Answer: X

What If the Condition Returns After Surgery?

The biggest concern after back surgery is a reoccurrence of the condition. The best result would be if the disease does not return. However there are too many cases in which patients do not show improvement following surgery. Surgery inevitably weakens the back. To perform surgery on a disc, an incision must be made on the surrounding muscles and ligaments. In order for the surgeon to approach the disc and nerves, a portion of the lamina must be removed. Eventually, spinal bones, as well as the muscles and ligaments surrounding the damaged disc, weaken due to surgery. Since the root causes are not addressed and just the protruding parts of the disc are excised during the surgery, there is always a possibility that the disc might re-rupture.

The real problem occurs when the disc ruptures again. Many doctors recommend another surgery when the disc re-herniates. The first surgery will have already weakened the spine and another surgery will further weaken it.

Success rates for re-operations are low. Therefore, discs that re-herniate must be treated with non-invasive methods that can strengthen the muscles and ligaments.

Answer: X

What If You Are Old with Diabetes, and Multiple Chronic Illnesses?

Many people contract chronic cardiovascular diseases such as diabetes, hypertension, and hyperlipidemia as they age. Because such people can suffer from excessive bleeding or delayed hemostasis during surgery, doctors do not recommend surgery for these patients even if they are suffering from lumbar spinal conditions. This makes certain back disc patients with spinal disorders think that there is no cure and to abandon treatment.

Mr. Kim, who visited Jaseng Hospital of Korean Medicine when he was about 80 years old, looked significantly older than his actual age. As in the case of other older adults, he also suffered from diabetes, cardiovascular disease, osteoporosis, and other health conditions. Due to his circumstances, a conventional medicine hospital had given up on treating him. In fact, conventional medicine doctors refrain from operating on people with diabetes because the disease can result in post-operative complications. The same is true for patients with osteoporosis, since performing back surgery on them can further weaken the vertebrae.

There is no need for patients to undergo surgery when there are too many potential surgical complications. Korean medicine's non-invasive treatments can be a good alternative that provides a high chance of success and recovery. In addition, Korean medicine non-invasive treatments strengthen the weakened body. Even for patients with other chronic conditions, certain treatments can still be implemented. Herbal medicine can be used to strengthen the bones and replenish energy while treating disc disease.

Various treatments can be combined to individualize an optimal program tailored to the individual patient.

Answer: X

What If You Have Herniated Discs in Both the Lumbar and Cervical Spine?

Patients with problems in their spine will likely experience both back and neck pain. These patients will likely experience pain in other joints. People who develop ruptured discs generally have congenitally weak spines, in addition to bad lifestyle, habits and posture. Since a combination of congenital factors and acquired causes weaken the discs, there is a high possibility that such people will suffer from both a cervical disc rupture and other spinal diseases.

In fact, patients who visit a hospital for lumbar disc herniation often return for cervical disc herniation later. That is why the initial treatment is important for disc herniation patients. Patients who receive surgery as their first treatment tend to repeatedly undergo surgery, which in turn will gradually harm their bodies further.

Surgery does not treat the fundamental causes of disc herniations, such as a congenital, physical, or bad lifestyles and habits. An operation only removes the symptoms of the disease. Since patients with multiple physical problems have multiple congenital and acquired conditions, their underlying conditions must be treated individually over the course of the program. That is the only way to prevent lumbar disc herniation from affecting other spinal diseases. Lumbar disc herniation treatment must also involve a wholesome approach in order to prevent cervical disc disease. The root causes of the condition, not just the symptoms, must be carefully addressed.

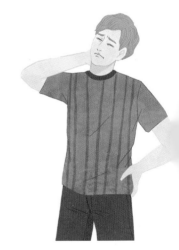

Answer: X

What If Your Symptoms Are Similar to Those of Others Who Had Herniated Disc Surgery?

Some patients ask, "I have a friend who underwent surgery. He and I have the same symptoms. That friend had good results from the surgery. He's still doing well today 10 years after the surgery. Don't you think I will also recover fully with surgery?"

Not all surgeries end up in failure. In many cases, surgeries are successful with good a prognoses. Failure is a distinct possibility as well. That is why the decision to operate must be made very carefully. In particular, stories of friends or acquaintances who have improved through surgery are not good reasons to undergo surgery yourself.

People have different physical constitutions. The pain might increase after surgery because the precise causes are not addressed during the operation, but the cause of increased pain might be the congenital physical constitution. Some people heal faster after surgery while others develop adhesions that press down on the nerves. People whose constitution makes them prone to developing adhesions will likely experience postoperative symptoms.

Since spinal surgery is a difficult procedure, it must take into consideration various physical constitutions and extra caution should be exercised. There is no guarantee that the good results your friends experienced will apply to you as well. If a patient remained healthy for 10 years after surgery, there is a possibility that the person's back was not in such a severe condition to begin with. It is highly likely that the patient could have stayed healthy for 20 to 30 years if he or she had received non-invasive treatment instead of surgery. The fact that the patient endured the weakened back conditions caused by surgery is proof that the person had a healthy back to begin with.

Rather than comparing yourself with other people, it is more important to know your own disc conditions and your physical constitution. The standard must always be yourself.

Answer: X

What If You Are Paralyzed and Cannot Move?

If the ruptured disc is severely compressing the nerves, causing paralysis, the patient can consider surgery. The paralysis that patients talk about is different from actual paralysis caused by a disc herniation. When patients say that they are paralyzed, what they really mean is that they cannot move because of their back pain. This is not true paralysis: It is only a temporary paralysis induced by our brain to prevent further damage to the ruptured discs in case of disc herniation.

Such temporary paralysis resolves within 7 to 10 days. Using emergency treatments such as Motion Style Acupuncture Treatment will enable temporarily paralyzed patients to move again within 30 minutes. True paralysis induced by a disc herniation is progressive, where the muscle strength of one leg is gradually lost. Such a condition may require surgery.

As such, doctors need to determine whether the paralysis is temporary or progressive. Patients who cite concerns for paralysis caused by disc herniation usually do not have true paralysis and do not need to undergo surgery. In most cases, the pain caused by a ruptured disc has induced the brain to protect the body by preventing its movements.

Motion Style Acupuncture Treatment can be an effective method to determine whether surgery is truly needed for in response to paralytic symptoms.

In cases of temporary paralysis, patients are able to start moving again in 30 minutes after receiving Motion Style Acupuncture Treatment. There are many cases in which patients who arrived in an ambulance because of paralytic symptoms recover within 30 minutes of receiving this type of treatment. Some patients have even been able to walk on their own to go to the bathroom. Korean medicine non-invasive treatments can sufficiently improve disc herniation symptoms within 1 to 2 weeks.

Answer: X

What If You Want a Quick Recovery?

Many disc patients seek to receive simple procedures or quick treatments because they wish to return to their daily routine as soon as possible. While some surgeries may appear simple, there are no simple operations. Any surgery requires the surgeon to damage the muscles before he or she can excise the protruded discs. With the popularization of surgeries using micrometer microscopes, surgical incisions have become much smaller. Smaller incisions still put a burden on the body. Because the incision is so small, there is not enough visibility is for the surgeon to maneuver under the skin more to operate on the damaged discs. Also, in some cases, surgeons need to drill a hole or excise a part of the vertebral bones.

As such, surgery can result in further back damage, which may delay the recovery process. Disc patients are prejudiced to think that Korean medicine treatment takes longer, but that is not the case. Two to 3 weeks of intensive inpatient treatments can induce quick recovery and return to daily activities.

Answer: X

What If You Have Bowel Obstruction?

Severe pain alone cannot determine whether a patient needs surgery. If severe pain continues for a long time, surgery might be required. However, if the pain gradually subsides through Korean medicine's non-invasive treatments, most patients will recover even without surgery.

The situation is different if the patient is suffering from urination or bowel movement issues. If the nerves controlling urination or bowel movement are affected in such a way that they prevent defecation or urination, the situation is likely to be urgent. The patient requires surgery, and the surgery must be conducted as soon as possible.

Answer: O

What If Pain Is Lasting Long After the Treatment?

Some patients who do not have severe pain consider whether they need surgery for a long time. Such patients tend to go in and out of treatment.

The most important thing about disc herniation treatment is not to follow the pain. Pain and disc herniation are two separate conditions. If the patient goes in and out of treatment depending on the pain level, the fundamental causes of disc herniation will not be treated, making the condition chronic.

Chronic disc herniation patients must seek a specialist who can provide continued care for their condition. Also, they need to consider receiving intensive treatment during a certain period. This is because such patients usually suffer from long-term pain, causing them to lose faith in their recovery.

These patients often seek treatment only at the beginning, and when they do not recover, they try to buy more time instead of handling the fundamental causes. Because they have been obsessing over the pain, the causes of the disease will worsen, making the treatment process more arduous. Those who are impatient about their symptoms should seek inpatient care to develop a belief that they can get better.

Answer: X

What If You Do Not Think the Treatment Will Be Effective Due to Your Old Age?

Many elderly patients say that their treatment will not be effective because of their advanced age. One elderly patient even said that he does not think he will get better because his bodily fluids are circulating no longer. Korean medicine has treatments, such as herbal medicine and pharmacopuncture, that seek to boost immunity and stimulate the body to produce more liquids. As such, Korean medicine treatments may be the best and safest option for elderly patients or patients with weaker physical constitutions.

Answer: X

What If You Cannot Control Your Pain Even with Painkillers?

Some patients complain about severe pain that does not subside even with painkillers. Since painkillers may lose their effectiveness and surgery might seem like a good option, but this is not the case. Such patients are well-suited for acupuncture treatment. Jaseng Hospital of Korean Medicine became well-known for its acupuncture treatment because it is much more effective than painkillers in reducing pain.

All around the world there have been many studies that compare the effects of analgesics and acupuncture treatment. In fact, even shallow-penetration acupuncture treatment is more effective than taking these medications. Since acupuncture has such a significant impact in controlling pain, acupuncture treatment can reduce the pain caused by lumbar disc herniation.

Answer: X

6

Nine Small But Important Questions Asked by Herniated Disc Patients

Q1

How Long Does It Take to Treat Herniated Discs?

Treatment Period Depends on the Condition of the Discs and the Patient

Before starting disc herniation treatment, many patients ask how long it will take for them to recover. The required duration of treatment depends on the state of the discs and that of the patient. Treatment methods can change depending on the disc condition; even the same treatment can have visible effects during different time periods for different patients.

Jaseng Hospital of Korean Medicine, however, does have specific standards that it uses to treating disc herniation. Two aspects should primarily be considered when treating disc conditions. The first aspect is the period of pain treatment, and the second aspect is the period of reinforcement treatment for the root causes of disc herniation.

The period will of course also depend on the condition of the patient. For example, even severe disc herniation can be quickly treated if the rate of nerve recovery is higher. However, a mild but chronic disc herniation may require a longer period to treat.

Although there are individual differences depending on the level of pain experienced by the patient, disc herniation pain can disappear as quickly as within 2 weeks of treatment.

In particular, if disc-induced inflammation dissipates quickly despite severe disc ruptures, pain can disappear as rapidly as within 2 weeks.

On the other hand, if disc herniation has been progressing for some time and the discs began degenerating, the patient might require long-term treatment lasting anywhere from 2 to 4 months. Chronic disc herniation patients experience duller pain than acute disc herniation patients do. However, because old and chronic pain does not subside easily, chronic disc herniation patients must receive treatment for the fundamental causes of their condition in addition to reinforcing treatments that strengthen adjoining areas.

Such reinforcing treatments can take at least 3 months. This is because damaged bones, nerves, muscles, and ligaments need at least 3 months to regenerate. That is, chronic disc herniation patients need to undergo reinforcement of treatment for at least 3 months even when their pain has resolved. In general, reinforcement treatment involves Chuna manual therapy that corrects posture, in addition to muscle reinforcement therapy.

Patients must also learn to manage their condition in their everyday lives. At Jaseng, during the first 2 months, patients learn good habits after treating the pain. Studies on disc herniation management recommend patients to continue their daily routine. Jaseng medical staff, however, recommend patients to postpone their daily routine while pain persists. Since patients are so sensitive to pain, they will think that their treatment has failed if they feel any pain as a result of straining their ruptured discs while performing daily tasks.

In reality, disc herniation does not relapse so easily from performing daily activities.

Even if a sudden strain causes sharp pain, the progress of the treatment does not disappear; such pain easily subsides. However, because the bodies and minds of patients undergoing disc herniation treatment are tired, they jump to the option of surgery even when they experience minor pain. That is why Jaseng recommends its patients to take care of themselves when participating in daily activities. This consequently helps to reduce the overall treatment period.

After pain treatments are completed, patients are taught to manage their conditions in everyday life. The medical staff teaches them how to properly use their muscles and how to exercise. Such a regimen must be maintained for at least 3 months. Because a habit takes about 3 months to become a routine, at least 3 months of practice are required for patients to build healthy habits for their back.

Some patients stop receiving treatment once their pain treatment is completed. Of course, each patient faces different circumstances, but patients who receive pain treatment followed by reinforcing treatment will generally have a better prognoses than those who stop seeing the doctor after a couple of months of pain treatment.

Patients who suspend their treatment after a couple of months do not fully understand back herniation and tend to only consider pain in relation to their disease. As such, when they return to their daily routines, they resume the bad habits that damages their discs, making them return to the hospital in just 1 or 2 years.

On the other hand, disc herniation will not reoccur for a long time for patients who continue treating the causes of their disc herniation even after their pain has subsided. In addition, because they learn about disc herniation from their doctor every time they visit the hospital, such patients will develop a thorough understanding of the features and management methods for disc herniation, which can help them practice good habits. Although their treatment periods are longer, since the possibility of relapse is smaller, they end up recovering more quickly.

Then, between a patient whose pain completely disappeared during treatment and a patient whose pain slightly remained, who will have a better prognosis? Ironically, patients with subtle, lingering pain after the treatment tend to have better prognoses.

Patients whose pain has completely disappeared tend to forget about the days in which they suffered from disc herniation, which induces them to also forget about the importance of back management they learned about during the course of their treatment. As the period of neglect continues, the disc herniation begins progressing again. Patients who have some remaining pain, however, will tend to remain cautious even after the treatment is completed. Such patients most likely continue practicing the spine management methods they learned during treatment, and actively work to avoid environments that can cause their discs to extrude. Such cases show that disc herniation is a disease that requires further management beyond pain treatment.

What Should I Do to Prevent the Conditions From Relapsing?

Proper Understanding of Discs

To prevent relapse of disc herniation, patients need to have proper knowledge of discs. Although it is not as prevalent in Korea, some other developed countries have what is called a "back school." These types of institutions teach people about back health. Medical professionals in some industrialized countries believe that management of disc herniation is the most important aspect of treatment, as treatment by itself can lead to repeated relapses. Back schools were established under the belief that management of the condition demands that patients properly understand the properties of the discs.

Back schools require patients to pay tuition. Numerous patients, however, gladly invest large amounts of money to receive the education. On the other hand, Korean patients rely only on medical professionals for information after paying their fees. Such attitudes must change quickly. Patients must develop a willingness to pay money to learn about back discs and ways to manage disc herniation symptoms.

As the old saying goes, back disc herniation patients must know their enemy well in order to avoid relapses. Patients who are knowledgeable about the properties of spinal discs understand that their diseases can progress even in the absence of immediate pain, and can be prepared for such occurrences.

People who know that disc herniation can easily progress under duress will make efforts to reduce the stress on their back and will think about how to use the back ergonomically, and what exercises will help their bodies.

As for exercises, acute disc herniation patients can benefit from isometric exercises. Isometric means that the lengths of the muscles do not change during the exercise. Examples include pushing against the wall. Bicep exercises contract the muscles, but on the other hand, pushing against the wall maintains the lengths of the muscles during the course of movement.

Strength training for muscles can cause the vertebral bones to move and stimulate the discs, which can also sprain the back. That is, while such exercises can strengthen the muscles, they may damage the discs. Isometric training, on the other hand, maintains the lengths of the muscles while strengthening them, keeping the spine protected. The downside of such exercises is that they cannot be conducted alone.

Therefore, patients must be educated about the mechanisms through which disc herniation develops, the current state of their disc conditions, and the types of exercises that are appropriate for them. Such education will enable the patients to receive more fundamental treatment and management, in addition to effectively preventing relapse.

I Already Have Data From Another Hospital. Why Do I Need Another Scan?

MRI Analysis Is More Important Than Scanning

MRI scanning is a sensitive issue that can cause misunderstandings between the patient and the hospital. Many patients think that hospital policy is designed in a way that forces them to take MRI scans. Other patients also believe that doctors recommend MRI scanning because the procedure is expensive. These are all not true. Analysis is more important than just scanning when it comes to MRI. In some cases, MRI images taken at another hospital can be difficult to analyze. If the images have been taken too long ago, or if the patient's symptoms have changed from what is indicated by the images, doctors will need new MRI images to accurately assess the patient's condition.

For hospitals, new MRI scans serve a defensive purpose. Many procedures are offered to patients these days. Some of these procedures that involve injections can cause spinal infections. They can also lead to tumors, which could be cancerous. These may not all show up in the MRI images that the patient provides.

A patient brought in MRI images that were 3 years old. Because the back symptoms from 3 years ago and the current symptoms did not seem very different and the MRI images explained the current pain, we decided not to take another round of images before beginning the treatment process.

But after some time, the doctor had a strange feeling and took new MRI images for the patient. Spinal tumors were discovered during the analysis. In cases like this, the patient may complain to the hospital about providing treatment for 3 months without knowing the precise cause of the illness. That is why many hospitals will require another round of MRI scanning that will reveal potential spinal infections and other diseases.

Q4

Can I Get Massages?

Non-Excessive Massages Are OK

Massages can be okay, but caution must be exercised. Disc herniation is a disease in which the discs are damaged and stimulate the nerves, which in turn induces pain in the muscles. This is why disc herniation is accompanied by myalgia.

Such pain can subside with light or warm massages that relaxes the muscles. As such, disc herniation patients should only receive soft massages that work on the superficial muscle layer. Some types of deep tissue massages compress the bones. Massages that go beyond the muscles – such as one in which the masseuse bends the back, steps on the back, or otherwise applies excessive force – can be harmful to disc herniation patients. Even when simply pressing down on the back, the masseuse must only massage the muscles, without compressing the bones.

Disc herniation can be worsened by the patient sneezing, or straining while on the toilet. In the same way, discs will be stimulated when abdominal pressure suddenly increases. The human body is a closed system. A sudden rise in abdominal pressure can impact and shock the discs. As such, while gentle oil massages that only touch the surface are fine, deep massages that apply excessive force should be avoided.

The posture in which disc herniation patients receive massages is also important. In general, massages are performed with the person lying prone. However, certain postures may be bad for disc herniation patients, particularly in the early stages of their conditions. In early-stage patients, lying down on their sides or holding something between their legs will induce a more comfortable posture. On the other hand, lying prone can make the back tense and stimulate the discs, thereby increasing the pain level.

Q5

Is It Better to Lie on the Floor or On the Bed?

It Depends On the Patient

In the past, it was said that disc patients should sleep on a hard floor rather than on a soft bed. In fact, beds did not use to have good mattress springs. Concaved mattresses tended to distort the S-line of the spine even further. The curve on the spine became even more curved when the patient laid down on a concave mattress, putting the spine in a crouched position. It is better for disc herniation patients to straighten out their backs, and a flexed position induced by a bad mattress can worsen the disc condition.

Today's mattresses, however, do not sag so much. Also, lying down on the hard floor can tense up the back even more. It is beneficial for lumbar disc herniation patients to sleep on a bed with good springs.

This, however, is only a general guideline. Disc herniation patients are advised to try out mattresses and choose the one that feels most comfortable. Different patients feel comfortable on different mattresses, depending on how their discs have herniated.

Overall, lying down on the back is the most comfortable position for most disc herniation patients, but some patients cannot sleep while lying down on their backs.

Such patients feel more pressure on their discs when lying down, and are forced to sleep in a seated position. During the acute stages of the disease, patients need to sleep in a position that compresses the discs the least. The body knows best what that position is. If the patient feels less pain in the back while lying down on the floor, that means that the patient should sleep on the floor. The same goes for beds. If the patient feels comfortable on a bed, that is the best sleeping surface for that patient. If it hurts, however, the patient should avoid it.

Q6

Can I Use the Handstanding Exercise Machine?
What Exercises Should I Do?

Handstanding Exercises Are Dangerous;
Walking Is Relatively Safe

Exercise is required to manage disc herniation conditions and prevent recurrence. Acute disc herniation, however, is different. The greatest risk factor in acute disc herniation is the patient choosing surgery due to severe pain. As such, acute disc herniation patients should rest at the early stages of the condition and refrain from exercising.

If the patient's condition is not acute, the best exercise is walking. Walking is the safest exercise within the scope allowed by disc herniation pain. Yoga and Pilates are two exercises in which disc herniation patients show the most interest. For people without disc herniation, both exercises are good for spinal health. This is because they extend the range of back movement.

People who exercise regularly have wider ranges of movement and better flexibility, in addition to having effective preventive methods that suit them. Their bodies also easily adapt to exercises. However, patients in their 40s and 50s who are diagnosed with early disc herniation should not suddenly start exercising excessively after a long period of immobility. Even healthy people will be easily injured if they begin bending their wrists 45 degrees when they usually bend them 15 degrees. When disc herniation patients suddenly begin exercising, their discs may be injured further and their initial disc conditions might worsen.

Disc patients also show interest in using an inversion machine. The basic principle for this exercise is that hanging upside down will reduce the top-to-bottom pressure on the discs, thereby relaxing the tense muscles. Of course, such effects do exist. Hanging upside down can relax the muscles and certainly make the patient feel more relaxed as well. This exercise forcefully relaxes the muscles, which is okay for people with healthy discs. However, those individuals with acute disc herniation symptoms should avoid this exercise, as it can excessively stimulate the damaged discs and muscles.

Since some physical therapy routines provide mild relaxation for isolated parts of the spine, we recommend that patients not to use the inversion machine while unsupervised at home. Also, the inversion machine forces the entire body to relax. Patients are advised to obtain an MRI at the hospital first, and then decide the level of the inversion exercise that will not place excessive stress on the body.

Sinyeon Therapy, a subset of Chuna manual therapy, uses the principles of the inversion exercise. Since there are ways to provide isolated relaxation for damaged discs, it is better to engage in therapy for such results. Inversion machines are discouraged not only for disc herniation patients, but also for degenerative disc patients.

Walking up the stairs is also okay for the back. Since walking does not put too much stress on the back, light walking is good for the spine. People with bad knee joints, however, do not benefit from walking up the stairs. Since people with bad back joints tend to have bad knee joints as well, such patients are recommended to walk on a flat surface rather than up the stairs.

The best exercise for the back is walking in water. Walking in water minimizes the pressure on the discs while providing significant exercise. Thus, it is perfect for disc herniation patients.

Q7

My Pain Keeps Traveling Between My Back and Hip. Is This Okay?

Traveling pain is an indication that the condition is not very serious.

People with really severe disc conditions do not say that their pain migrates. Patients with really severe symptoms point to a specific area of pain. They say which areas hurt and when they hurt more. More serious disc herniation symptoms will lead the patients to more precisely point out specific pain areas. In such patients, damaged discs compress specific nerves, allowing them to know exactly which areas are experiencing pain.

When they are treated and the symptoms subside, they say something like the following:

"In the past, my right leg was pulling back as it hurt. Now, my right leg is okay but my left leg seems to hurt as well. Or it might be my back. It feels like my pain is moving around."

It is not really a bad thing that the pain is migrating around the body. If there is a serious problem in one spot, only that part hurts because the brain only recognizes pain in that area. When the pain travels around, however, it means that the damage is not serious enough. It is in fact easier to treat the disease if the pain is migrating around the body. When this happens, the pain may subside even without treatment. Migratory pain is also part of the process of resolving pain.

However, the migrating pain can be caused because of overall distortion and imbalance in the body. As such, it should always not be seen as a good sign. It may also mean that the damage is present in multiple locations and appropriate treatment is required. It is necessary to accurately identify the cause of migratory pain to provide appropriate treatment.

Q8

What Conditions Should I Watch for?

Changes in the Senses Must Be Monitored

First of all, pain is not a symptom that should be watched for. Since pain ebbs and flows in the healing process, it is not a signal of risk. Pain simply indicates the progress of healing.

A more serious physical sensation that indicates abnormalities in the body is any change in any of the senses. When discs pop out significantly, they may compress the nerves that control urination and bowel movement, causing cauda equina syndrome and a resulting change in the senses. Since only 1 out of 10,000 people suffers from cauda equina syndrome, it is a relatively uncommon disease.

Cauda equina syndrome patients begin experiencing abnormal urination and bowel movements, in addition to a gradual loss of muscle strength. Even with such symptoms, improvement or maintenance of such lowered muscle strength can be a good sign. However, patients should take note if muscle strength continues to deteriorate.

In rare cases, muscle strength may deteriorate while pain levels subside. Assuming that unbearable pain is a level 10, most patients' pain level decrease to a 5 or 6 after 2 to 3 weeks of treatment. If patients suddenly experience loss of muscle strength and cannot use their muscles well, there is a high possibility that surgery is indicated. But because such changes in the senses and muscle strength cannot be easily detected by the patient, the doctor must continue checking for such signs.

Q9

Why Do I Experience Significantly More Pain at Night?

There are varying and conflicting opinions regarding why some patients experience more pain at night. In Korean medicine, patients with more blood stasis will experience more pain at night. When disc results in damage to the surrounding tissues, blood stasis, or "dead blood," can build up in that region. A physiological phenomenon that tries to remove the pooling blood will cause pain in the body. Because such processes are partially more active at night, the pain is more pronounced at night. This is called blood stasis pain.

Also, because people feel psychologically isolated from the external environment at night, they tend to think more about their internal pain. That might be the reason that disc herniation patients feel their pain more acutely at night. Even common dental pains can be forgotten when we watch interesting TV programs. In the same manner, we are less sensitive to pain during the day because our minds are occupied with other things, while that is not necessarily the case at night. Such explanations, however, are not sufficient. Since cancerous pain and other pains accompanying serious problems worsen at night, doctors always pay special attention to nocturnal pain. This is an area that requires more research.

References

- Hirabayashi S,KumanoK, Tsuiki T, Eguchi M, Ikeda S: A dorsally displaced free fragment of lumbar disc herniation and its interesting histologic findings. A case report. Spine 15:1231–1233, 1990.

- Slavin KV, Raja A, Thornton J, Wagner FC Jr: Spontaneous regression of a large lumbar disc herniation: report of an illustrative case. Surg Neurol 56:333–336, 2001.

- Doita M, Kanatani T, Ozaki T, Matsui N, Kurosaka M, Yoshiya S: Influence of macrophage infiltration of herniated disc tissue on the production of matrix metalloproteinases leading to disc resorption. Spine 26:1522–1527, 2001.

- Henmi T, Sairyo K, Nakano S: Natural history of extruded lumbar intervertebral disc herniation. J Med Invest 49:40–43, 2002.

- Ahn SH, AhnMW, ByunWM: Effect of the transligamentous extension of lumbar disc herniations on their regression and the clinical outcome of sciatica. Spine 25:475–480, 2000.

- Maigne JY, Rime B, Deligne B: Computed tomographic follow-up study of forty-eight cases of nonoperatively treated lumbar intervertebral disc herniation. Spine 17:1071–1074, 1992.

- Virri J, Grönblad M, Seitsalo S, et al. Comparison of the prevalence of inflammatory cells in subtypes of disc herniations and associations with straight leg raising. Spine26:2311–5,2001

- Tamer Orief, Yasser Orz, Walid Attia, Khaled Almusrea:Spontaneous Resorption of Sequestrated Intervertebral Disc Herniation. Spine journal World Neurosurg 77,1:146–152,2012

- Chung HJ, Lee HS, Shin JS, Lee SH, Park BM, Youn YS, et al. Modulation of acute and chronic inflammatory processes by a traditional medicine preparation GCSB-5 both in vitro and in vivo animal models. J Ethnopharmacol. 2010;130(3):450–459.

- Kim TH, Yoon SJ, Lee WC, Kim JK, Shin J, Lee S, et al. Protective effect of GCSB-5, an herbal preparation, against peripheral nerve injury in rats. J Ethnopharmacol. 2011;136(2):297–304.

- Kim JK, Park SW, Kang JW, Kim YJ, Lee SY, Shin J, et al. Effect of GCSB-5, a Herbal Formulation, on MonosODIum Iodoacetate-Induced Osteoarthritis in Rats. Evid Based Complement Alternat Med. 2012;2012:730907.

- Park Y-G, Ha C-W, Han C-D, Bin S-I, Kim H-C, Jung Y-B, et al. A prospective, randomized, double-blind, multicenter comparative study on the safety and efficacy of Celecoxib and GCSB-5, dried extracts of six herbs, for the treatment of osteoarthritis of knee joint. Journal of ethnopharmacology. 2013;149(3):816–24.

- Effects of intra-articular SHINBARO treatment on monosodium iodoacetate-induced osteoarthritis in rats.Kim WK, Chung HJ,./Chin Med

- Comparison of EQ-5D index values for NeuP and common chronic diseases. Abbreviations: ALS, amyotrophic lateral sclerosis; DN, diabetic neuropathy; FBSS, failed back surgery syndrome; MND, motor neurone disease; NeuP, neuropathic pain; NYHA, New York Heart Association; PD, Parkinson's disease; PHN, post-herpetic neuralgia

- A study on the causes of failed back syndrome and the treatment performances. Kim BJ. Journal of Korean Society of Spine Surgery. 1999;6(1):135–40.

- The multiply operated lumbar spine. Wiesel SW. Instr Course Lect. 1985;34:68–83.

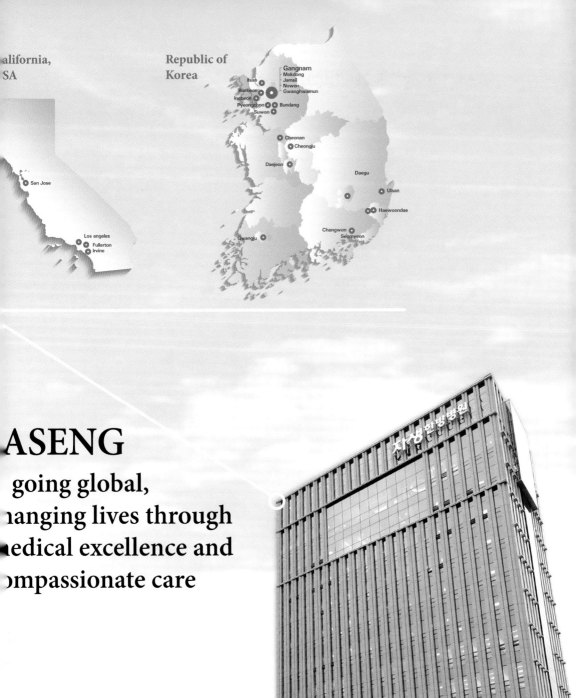

California,
USA

San Jose

Los angeles
Fullerton
Irvine

Republic of
Korea

Ilsan
Bucheon
Incheon
Pyeongchon   Bundang
Suwon

Gangnam
Mokdong
Jamsil
Nowon
Gwanghwamun

Cheonan
Cheongju

Daejeon

Daegu

Ulsan

Haewoondae

Changwon
Seomyeon

Gwangju

ASENG

going global,
hanging lives through
medical excellence and
ompassionate care

Jaseng in Gangnam, Seoul

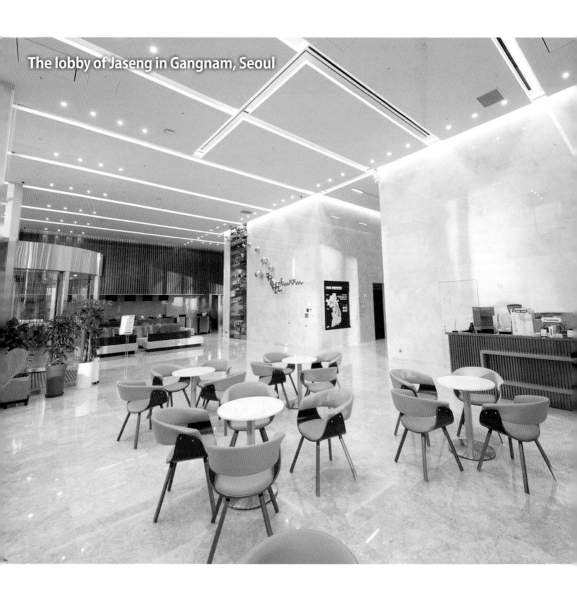

The lobby of Jaseng in Gangnam, Seoul

Over 900 medical staff working full-time to provide highest quality non-invasive spinal treatments to patients as the largest spine-specialty hospital in Korea equipped with 1,394 inpatient beds.